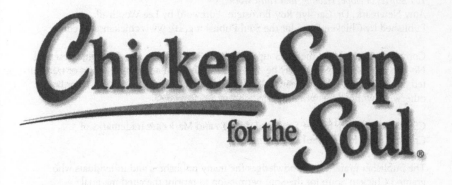

Chicken Soup for the *Soul*®

Recovering from Traumatic Brain Injuries

Chicken Soup for the Soul: Recovering from Traumatic Brain Injuries
101 Stories of Hope, Healing, and Hard Work
Amy Newmark, Dr. Carolyn Roy-Bornstein. Foreword by Lee Woodruff
Published by Chicken Soup for the Soul Publishing, LLC www.chickensoup.com

Front cover photo courtesy of iStockPhoto.com/jjneff (© John Neff).
Interior photo courtesy of iStockPhoto.com/LdF (© LdF).

Cover and Interior Design & Layout by Brian Taylor, Pneuma Books, LLC

Distributed to the booktrade by Simon & Schuster. SAN: 200-2442

Publisher's Cataloging-in-Publication Data
(Prepared by The Donohue Group)

Chicken soup for the soul : recovering from traumatic brain injuries :
  101 stories of hope, healing, and hard work / [compiled by] Amy Newmark
  [and] Dr. Carolyn Roy-Bornstein ; foreword by Lee Woodruff.

     pages ; cm

     ISBN 978-1-61159-938-1

     1. Brain damage--Patients--Rehabilitation--Literary collections. 2. Brain
  damage--Patients--Rehabilitation--Anecdotes. 3. Brain--Wounds and injuries--
  Patients--Rehabilitation--Literary collections. 4. Brain--Wounds and injuries--Patients-
  -Rehabilitation--Anecdotes. 5. Anecdotes. I. Newmark, Amy. II. Roy-Bornstein,
  Carolyn. III. Woodruff, Lee. IV. Title: Recovering from traumatic brain injuries

RC387.5 .N87 2014
617.4/810443/02   2014934627

PRINTED IN THE UNITED STATES OF AMERICA
on acid∞free paper

24 23 22   08 09 10

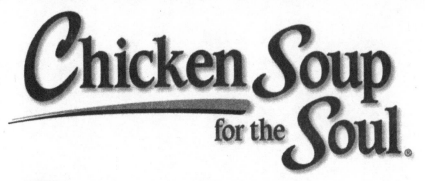

Chicken Soup for the Soul®
Recovering from Traumatic Brain Injuries

101 Stories of Hope, Healing, and Hard Work

Amy Newmark
Dr. Carolyn Roy-Bornstein
Foreword by Lee Woodruff

Chicken Soup for the Soul Publishing, LLC
Cos Cob, CT

Chicken Soup for the Soul

www.chickensoup.com

Contents

❶

~But You Look So Normal~

❷

~Self-Discovery~

❸

~Never Giving Up~

❹

~Healing Power of Mother Nature~

5

~Acceptance~

6

~A Family Affair~

❼

~Attitude Is Everything~

❽

~Coping Strategies that Work~

❾

~Opportunity Knocks~

⑩

~Making a Difference~

~Making a Difference~

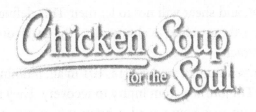

Foreword

I t's hard for me to imagine that there was a point in my life when I had no idea what TBI meant. *Traumatic Brain Injury.* That diagnosis is as devastating, complicated, individual and scary as any that can be delivered in the medical profession.

There are no percentages, no miracle cures, no accurate ways to predict how well someone will or will not recover. There is no time-table for when they will wake up from a coma and no way to assess what they will be left with in terms of "their old self."

Having a TBI, or being connected to someone who has suffered one, is an exercise in extreme patience. The slow process of recovery makes "watching paint dry" feel like the speed of light. Yes, it's that slow.

Which is why I had to put my "Type A" just-get-it-done person-ality aside and accept that we didn't have any control over this one. Waiting for Bob to wake up from his coma, and then watching him regain his words and cognition, was a very clear reminder that none of us have our hands on the script for how life goes.

In those weeks and months, and throughout that first year of my husband's recovery, I taught myself to truly take things day by day, and even at some points, hour by hour. Navigating myself, my family and our extended families through Bob's brain injury taught me some of my most important lessons in life. And you'll find many of those life lessons in the pages of this book, written by the amazing men and women who have walked in similar shoes. And while every one of these journeys is a little bit different, the sense of resilience, determination and sheer will not to let their TBIs define them is one of the amazing things I find in almost all of the survivors with whom I come in contact.

The compendium of stories here, 101 in all, illuminate the many facets of the TBI journey, from injury to recovery. They are a wonderful testament to just how varied a brain injury can be. They also highlight that element of human nature that is hardwired to look for the gift and the positive transformations that come in the wake of disaster and tragedy.

This book is a wonderful bridge between the military TBI community and the civilian one. While I spend a large part of my time with military families, I recognize the stories in this book—they are the same loving, heartbreaking, familiar ones that I hear from our returning service members. While our veterans are largely wounded by acts of war, the civilian injuries happen in the same "in an instant" way, whether it's car accidents, falls, or something as simple as a door opening suddenly in someone's face. It's stunning how so many people experience a permanent, life-altering TBI from something mundane. You'll read about one woman who got her TBI when she and her young daughter knocked heads while horsing around.

In the span of years since Bob's injury, there are days I feel like I have become a virtual expert on traumatic brain injuries, at least to the extent that one can become an expert on one of the least understood parts of the human body. I am blessed that many folks want to share their stories with me. After the publication of our book, *In an Instant*, Bob and I find ourselves on the receiving end of phone calls from frantic loved ones, we get manuscripts relating other people's amazing TBI stories, and we are often asked to talk to groups about our experiences. We do as much as we can, and I am particularly excited about writing the foreword for this book because stories are of paramount importance. It was the stories of the survivors and the thrivers after TBI that kept me going during the very dark moments of our own experience, the times when I didn't know what would become of our little family. Stories connect us, they show us the commonality of experience and they inspire us; they help us to understand that if someone else could find their way, we can too.

How did I get here? How did we become, at least for a time, the national poster family for TBI?

On January 29, 2006, I joined the club that no one wants to be a member of—the more than 2.5 million families every year, just in the United States, who receive the devastating news that their loved one has suffered from traumatic brain injury. I went from a working mother of four with a full life to an overnight caregiver, sitting by a bedside wondering if my husband would live or die. I went from expecting my TV-anchor husband to be able to deliver the news from any location with his photographic memory to hoping that he would simply emerge from his coma and remember who we were.

Let me back up. Because every story has a before and after and it's only in the aftermath of any traumatic and life-altering event that we truly understand all of the many things we were taking for granted—just assuming would always be there. TBIs have a way of reorganizing your priorities instantly and a way of changing your worldview.

After more than a decade at ABC News, covering just about every major story out there, Bob was named co-anchor of ABC's *World News* after Peter Jennings' sad and untimely death from lung cancer. Bob and Elizabeth Vargas were going to take ABC into the next generation of news.

Just six weeks after taking the anchor chair, Bob was reporting from Iraq for what was his eighth trip there. He had been embedded with the marines during the invasion of Iraq and had covered wars for over a decade. When he would leave to report from areas of conflict, while I certainly didn't dwell on it, I knew that his job called for him to be in dangerous situations. I understood he could be shot, or be in a car accident, or be kidnapped—all of these scenarios usually involved death at worst, or physical injury or disability at least. But not once did I consider the possibility of a head injury. In fact, I had never really known anyone who'd suffered a head injury.

What happened to Bob on that January day, on a dusty road

in Balad, Iraq, is what had been happening and still happens to our troops and innocent civilians in the wars in Iraq and Afghanistan every single day. Driving down a road, halfway out of a tank, a 125 millimeter roadside bomb was detonated about twenty-five feet from where Bob was taping a news "stand up" over the roar of the engine. The explosion was powerful enough to shatter Bob's skull on the left side and send his helmet soaring hundreds of yards away, forever changing the trajectory of all our lives.

What happened next is the stuff of heroism. It is the thing that can often make the difference in outcome for those with TBIs, because time is of the essence to treat and release pressure from a rapidly swelling brain.

It was the quick acting and very brave military team around Bob who did not hesitate. It was the medics who ignored the order not to land the helicopter in the midst of a gunfight. They got Bob and his cameraman out of the battle zone without any concern for their own lives. It was the doctors, nurses and medics who, despite operating on a military base where the "hospital" was fashioned out of tents and run on generators, with doctors and nurses wearing full body armor, continued to saw sixteen centimeters of Bob's skull off while they were taking mortar fire. That's right, did you get that last part? They were taking mortar fire while they were operating on my husband and they just kept going. The men and women who volunteer to serve their country have my utmost respect and admiration. They are there on the battlefield so that the rest of us can have choices about joining the military, and they are my personal heroes. No matter what your politics, we all owe our veterans a debt of gratitude.

There is no question that fast action and the understanding of head trauma were critical factors in that golden hour of medicine. That exceptional and timely medical care is certainly a big part of the reason that Bob is back with us as a father, husband, and a journalist who has re-taken the stage of his own life in ways that make me tear up even as I write this.

Bob was taken to the military hospital in Baghdad, transferred to Landstuhl, Germany and then brought to Bethesda Naval Hospital in Washington by air transport, all within seventy-two hours. He was back home in the States before I could even begin processing that this was us—this was our family—my husband had been hit by a bomb and they believed he had taken shrapnel to the brain. My husband had a traumatic brain injury.

After thirty-six days in a medically-induced coma, Bob woke up, very suddenly, without the usual slower transition that most experience. He was happy and loving, funny and very grateful to be alive. Practically every doctor and nurse in that hospital came in to witness the miracle of his abrupt awakening. Bob was missing words, easily fatigued and working hard to try to put the pieces back together. I began to understand, as the initial euphoria wore off, that this was going to be a long haul. We were getting ready to embark on the old "this is a marathon not a sprint" journey. That is a clichéd inside-TBI phrase I really learned to hate!

If I had thought that Rehabilitation would hold some secrets or silver bullets, I was wrong. It came down to day-to-day hard work and repetition, the determination of my husband to get back to himself—to do that for me, for our four children and of course, for himself. Watching him make that journey, from trying to relearn Mandarin Chinese in the hopes that it would improve his English, to painstakingly undergoing writing exercises, was inspiring and humbling. I fell in love with him even more as I witnessed his sheer determination to triumph.

During our six weeks in the military hospital, we had the privilege of meeting many young men and women and their families on the TBI ward. We watched the different scenarios in the rooms around us: the service members with close families, the ones whose spouses could not afford to leave the children and come to the bedside in DC for long periods, the very young couples, the mothers caretaking sons, most with limited resources. It was in those moments, realizing how lucky we were with our own wonderful network of friends and family and the support of Bob's employer, Disney-ABC, that we decided we would use our voices to bring attention to our brain-injured service members. We understood that attention would also spill over into the civilian world of brain injury, which I would come to learn was one of the most underfunded, neglected areas of the health care spectrum.

The journey we made by founding the Bob Woodruff Foundation was part of the silver lining for our family, the chance to raise money and awareness for our military families and to try to ease the road for others, after understanding the hurdles that get put in the way with this often frustrating and elusive invisible injury.

That's why we are so grateful that this important book will not only help TBI survivors and their families navigate their way through the recovery process, providing them with emotional support, understanding, and a sense of community, but also that proceeds from this book's sales will help our Foundation do its work. We thank Chicken Soup for the Soul for this contribution to the TBI community.

As so many of these wonderful stories illustrate, TBIs are so difficult, because unlike an obvious injury, the outside world doesn't know anything is wrong. Many of these stories have come more to the fore with the tremendous number of head injuries from the recent wars in Iraq and Afghanistan. The legacy of these wars will be the more than 360,000 service members who have received some form of a brain injury—whether it's a visible TBI wound from direct injury or the invisible internal wounds of multiple concussive blasts, post-traumatic stress or combat stress. Many of these soldiers wouldn't have survived their head wounds in previous wars, or would have been diagnosed with "shell shock" and written off by society, living in "the back of the house," as one doctor described it to me. But today we continue to discover more about the brain and how to help it heal. You will see many wonderful examples of healing in the stories on these pages.

The great number of brain injuries, the signature injury of these wars, has also helped to bring attention to TBI in general and shine a light on how we protect our athletes from concussions and TBIs. More attention is being paid to athlete safety, from the middle school field to the professional arena, and also to post-concussion care for athletes. All of this is important to help guide future rules and laws and behaviors in the area of prevention.

It was a full year before I let my breath out with Bob. A full year before I allowed myself to believe that this was all headed in a good direction, that he, and we, might be okay. During that time I had many balls in the air, making sure the kids were okay, getting back to work, supporting Bob's recovery. I was Bob's advocate, his nurse, his best friend and his protector. And in that first year especially, it was an adjustment to shift the relationship back from being a full-time caregiver to more of a wife and partner as he began to recover.

I learned many things on this unexpected journey with TBI. I learned the beauty of being more in the present. That sounds like a greeting card line, but in the absence of being able to do anything else, I had to face each day with my own inner sense of peace, filter out the negative I didn't want to deal with and try to focus on what was right in front of me to remain hopeful. Looking ahead too far down the road was scary and sometimes looking back was sad, so I learned to love exactly where I was in the moment. I've tried to adopt this outlook in the way I live now, even though it's not possible every single day.

Speaking of hope, I learned that with a TBI, many folks, especially in the acute care stage, believe it's their job to minimize your expectations, to circumscribe your loved one's chances for recovery so that you don't get "your hopes up." I tried not to listen to those people. I wasn't going to let anyone beat anything out of me that might help me to get through each day; to keep Bob and my family feeling positive and upbeat, to give me the energy to put my feet on the floor each day and walk in the ICU. I didn't want anyone to rush to judgment about my husband's prognosis, especially before he had woken up. In those early days, I was determined to understand TBI on my terms, without going on the Internet and scaring the pants off myself. When all we could do was wait and pray, I needed to leave room for hope to be nuanced, for me to believe that my husband might be the recipient of a miracle. Why not? I have come to understand that hope can be found even in terminal situations. Hope doesn't have to mean cure. But it should always allow for wonderful, loving and appropriate care.

I learned firsthand that no one successfully gets through any big event without some combination of what I call the 4 F's: family, friends, faith and funny. That last one, a sense of humor, is critical to living in the land of TBI. You'd better be able to laugh together and as a family if you are going to survive the very long stretch between injury and recovery. Bob and I have numerous examples of funny moments where we all cracked up. Laughter heals; it releases good things, so learn to laugh together. It sure beats crying. Gallows humor came about for a very practical reason. When you whistle past the graveyard and laugh at the thing that scares you, you remove some of the power it has over you.

And finally, I have come to understand that recovery is a continuum. You never are "fully healed," in the sense that you will return to exactly who you were before the injury. But the good news is that the brain continues to repair itself years and decades after the injury. I remember Trisha Meili, the "Central Park Jogger," telling me that all of these years later after her attack, she still sees improvements. Our brains—with their astounding neuroplasticity and ability to recover and reconnect—are a surprising source of good news and inspiration for all the families who live with brain injury. And as Bob says, "We are constantly changing and growing and transforming as humans. We never remain the exact same person we were, TBI or not."

I know that we are among the lucky ones. We had excellent medical care right off the bat, we had the best resources, and often, when Bob's progress could have gone one way or the other, it went the right way. It also helped that Bob had such a good attitude. When he woke up from his coma, I was worried he would be depressed, as is common among TBI patients at various points. After all, he had just started his dream job at the apex of his career and then, six weeks later, it was taken away by a bomb—in an instant.

But instead of asking "Why me?" Bob said, "Why not me? What makes me any different or more special than the twenty-five-year-old kid from Kansas who is sitting in a tank. Just because I'm on TV?"

That was the moment I decided if he wasn't going to feel sorry for himself, then that was the way I would choose to move through the world. I can't tell you we both didn't experience sorrow and loss and grief—that's part of the process—but that outlook did make a huge difference in Bob's recovery and mine. Many marriages do not make it through the TBI journey. I am thankful that ours remained as strong as ever.

As you read this collection of personal, revealing stories, you'll take a journey through the world of TBI—reading about the myriad ways that people suffer their TBIs, the ups and downs of recovery, and the new paths our writers have followed since their TBIs. Some people were in comas for a long time; others weren't even diagnosed with their TBIs until years after they occurred, having been told it was "just a concussion." You'll read stories from family members about their roles as caregivers and cheerleaders, advice from healthcare professionals, and you'll pick up great tips from caregivers and from the patients themselves, coping strategies that may work for you too.

You'll also read a lot about accepting a new normal, finding the good in the bad, and working hard. Persistence, positive thinking, and perspective are key themes throughout the book. The stories are inspiring and motivating, a great boost for your spirit, as well as a source of information. You'll undoubtedly find some stories that particularly resonate with you that you'll return to over and over again.

I need to make one final comment before I set you off on your own journey of healing, comfort, and community through these 101 stories. And that is that nothing will ever be the same again. I love the fact that most of the stories in this book are written by the person with the TBI. So you can meet the survivors, hear about their recoveries, and develop an understanding of how their lives are permanently changed. Many abandoned their original careers, or embarked on new ones they like even more. Many talk about their permanent impairments. But many also talk about the gifts they have found in their new lives.

I hope that this book not only helps all of the TBI patients and their families out there, but also raises awareness of the TBI issue in the civilian and military population. The next time you are frustrated by someone slowly counting out change in the grocery store line ahead of you, remember you may be standing behind a TBI survivor. Maybe even someone who raised his hand when his country asked him to go. There are millions of TBI survivors out there. And they are all the bravest, most resilient people I know.

~Lee Woodruff

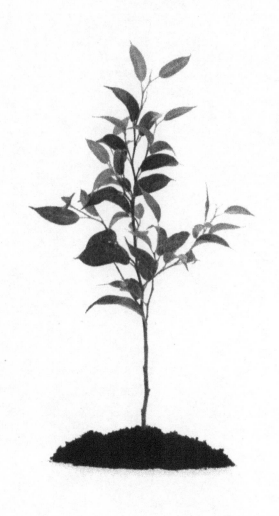

Chapter 1

Recovering *from* Traumatic Brain Injuries

But You Look So Normal

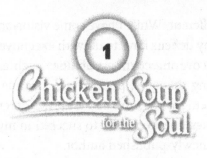

As I Am Now

*I now see how owning our story and loving ourselves through that process is
the bravest thing that we will ever do.*

~Brené Brown

"You look fine. Are you sure you're hurt? How did you injure your head anyway?" I'd like to say that I broke my brain doing a cool flip while waterskiing, or something fun like that. Pretty much anything would be better than the truth: I'm a klutz.

It was a blustery January day in Michigan, when a day of freezing rain was followed by a day of heavy snow. Early in the afternoon, I drove to a convenience store to pick up snacks for what I expected to be a long night at the office. As I walked back to my car, I slipped on some ice and smacked my head on the concrete. I don't know if I passed out, or if I did, for how long. I don't know if anyone saw me or tried to help me. At some point, I got up... and drove home.

My townhouse was only a mile away. I called a colleague and uttered some nonsense that drew her concern. She ignored my insistence that I felt fine and drove me to the emergency room. I told the doctor there that I felt fine, too. So while they X-rayed my arm, they didn't do a CT scan of my brain. My arm was put in a sling and my brain and I were sent home to rest. I was told to follow up with my regular doctor.

The next day I woke up with an excruciating headache and an unwelcome initiation to the world of traumatic brain injury. Every brain injury is different. While I have some vision and balance issues, the majority of my deficits have to do with executive function, which is a broad term covering cognitive abilities such as memory, multi-tasking, organizing thoughts, prioritizing, time management, recalling details, problem solving, and initiating and executing projects. In short, all the things I needed to do to succeed in my job as a marketing director and newly-published author.

When I first ventured out of my home, I realized that a healthy brain filters out sounds and sights so that one can focus on what is needed at the moment. An injured brain can't do that. When I returned to work a few weeks after my injury, and against the advice of my neurologist, I was overwhelmed by the cacophony of sounds: multiple radios on multiple stations, multiple conversations with multiple voices. All the noises jumbled together at the level of a rock concert; I was amazed anyone could get anything done. The lights seemed brighter too, so I looked for my sunglasses. Any movement seemed lightning fast and I was disoriented. I plopped in my chair and promptly fell to the floor. My sense of balance was out of whack as well. In my confusion I became aware of another sensation: nausea. I made it to the bathroom just in time. A coworker drove me home. I sat in the silence of my home wondering what had just happened to my life.

The first three years were the most difficult. I just couldn't comprehend that I would never successfully work again. I might have a few good weeks, then I'd spend the next two in bed. Even more unsettling, I would have periods where I thought I was doing well, but people told me that I was speaking gibberish. I would get so frustrated that they couldn't understand me, not aware that what I was saying was not understandable. As someone who had always persevered through challenges, it seemed utterly counterintuitive that the worst thing I could do now was push myself too hard. My recovery was marked by many periods of hopeful progress, followed by soul-crushing setbacks.

When things were going well, friends who knew the old me would start to inquire about when I'd start writing again. I realize that people meant well, but the reality is that I have permanent brain damage. Permanent. While I may get glimpses of that old creative spark, I can't maintain it. It's like my brain used to be a souped-up Jaguar. Now it's a broken-down jalopy. I might still be able to get from point A to point B, but the ride is a lot different now, and while the Jag is just getting started, the junker is headed back to the shop.

People have this idea that if you have a disability, you are only as good as your worst day. I do have plenty of bad days. But I do have good days, too. I've noticed these come when I've avoided the things that trigger my symptoms, like crowds and stressful situations. Occasionally I have great days and feel like my old self. But I am always aware that I can't take my health for granted.

The losses I've faced are significant, if not visible. My family and friends know that I can never offer a definitive RSVP. Each day is a new lottery. Will it be a rare good day when I can be productive and play catch-up? Will it be yet another fair day when I choose my priorities and let my rock-steady husband pick up the slack? Or will it be a bad day when snuggling my son all day in my quiet, dark bed is the best that I can do?

A couple years after my injury, when I was in the throes of self-pity, I had a chance conversation with a colleague at a conference. After pouring out my frustrations and fears, his response freed me from the futile hope of ever returning to my old life and gave me the grace to accept whatever the future might bring. He told me the following:

May you experience joy... as you are now
May you have peace with yourself... as you are now
May you have patience with yourself... as you are now
May you show kindness to yourself... as you are now
May you seek the goodness in yourself... as you are now
May you renew faithfulness in your life... as you are now
May you show gentleness to yourself... as you are now
May you exhibit self-control in your thoughts toward yourself...
as you are now

May you love yourself... as you are now.

His words became my mantra as I clawed my way back from depression. They stayed with me as I met and married my husband. They formed the basis of how I see myself now as a parent. Ten years ago, I was a Type-A single career woman. Today I am a Type-Z stay-at-home mom. I like to think I am a kinder, more accepting person now. My brain injury has made me realize my need for grace. And I am more willing to extend grace to others... as they are now. I'm more willing to give people the benefit of the doubt because I know that the outside doesn't always show what's going on inside. Though my head is still injured, my heart is healthier than ever.

~Jen Abbas de Jong

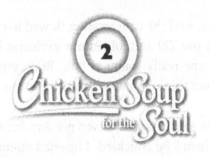

I Have a Secret

Not all those who wander are lost.

~J.R.R. Tolkien

I have a secret. Not all is as it appears. Most anyone living with a traumatic brain injury already knows this. We've all heard someone say "but you look normal," and we know that person doesn't get it.

I live in the new "Frontier Land" that is life with a brain injury. We can even spot each other. About a year after my brain injury, a new man appeared strolling in my neighborhood. He was a bit older than me. He walked with a cane and his wife ever present by his side.

As I still cycle twenty-five miles a day through our neighborhood streets, I know most of the local regulars by sight. I have given most of them oddball nicknames like "Dog-walking Lady" and "The Power Walking Couple."

My wife Sarah and I drove past this new neighbor regularly. Month by month, we could see his pace increasing and his stability improving. "I bet he had a brain injury," Sarah guessed.

Quite unexpectedly, I found myself stopped at a corner on my bike as the man and his wife walked by one day. The dis-inhibition that comes with brain injury can be so freeing. My first words brought huge smiles to them both.

"You are doing so well. It's great to see the progress you've made." Introductions were shared, though his name, like so many others, is forever lost to me. And the conversation flowed like water. He fell on ice the year after my TBI and joined our exclusive brain injury club, the one that no one really wants to join. Brain injury is indeed the last thing you ever think about—until it's the only thing you think about.

"The doctors said I would never get any better, but I decided not to listen to them," he chuckled. I listened intently to his tale and smiled.

Then I dropped my own verbal bomb. "My brain injury was a year before yours and like you, my own doctor said I was permanently disabled and to not expect much. I didn't listen either!" We shared a hale and hearty laugh and went our respective ways.

And my secret? My TBI has taught me that all is not as it appears. That old man fumbling with his wallet in front of me at the checkout counter no longer makes me impatient. He might be someone affected by traumatic brain injury. That driver cruising along at ten miles per hour under the posted speed limit no longer makes me tap my foot. She might be one of the 5.3 million people in the U.S. living with a disability from a traumatic brain injury. The person at the supermarket with his shopping cart parked dead center in the aisle as he stares at all the soups? You know where I am going with this. We are everywhere.

My TBI continues to teach me a level of patience, understanding and compassion I never had before my accident. When someone passes by you and does something you didn't quite expect, remember that they might just be one of us. After all, we look normal.

~David A. Grant

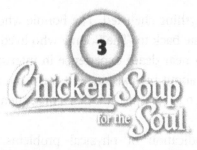

Forgiving Myself

Your pain is the breaking of the shell that encloses your understanding.

—Khalil Gibran

On November 18, 1979, a van traveling over seventy-five miles per hour crashed into my Volkswagen bug and pushed it across three lanes of traffic into a telephone pole. The driver never applied the brakes. The officer on scene said that if my gas tank had contained more than fumes my car would have exploded. I was in a coma, had a broken back, a collapsed lung, and the potential for multiple other internal injuries. The doctor told my mother to gather family, that I was in God's hands, and even if I lived through the night, I would never again live independently. He told her to go ahead and make funeral arrangements.

After only two weeks in the hospital, it was decided that I was well enough to go home. Ignoring the advice of my neurologist, I went off to college less than two months later. I never gave my neurologist a chance to explain the seriousness of my injuries, nor how those injuries might affect my future. I was in full blown denial, never understanding that denial after traumatic brain injury is defined as the inability of the brain to compare the difference between behavior and abilities before the injury, and behavior and abilities afterward.

The accident was not only the pivotal point between the safe cocoon of high school and life on my own. It was also the pivotal point between the Bonnie I knew, who died, and the Bonnie I lived to be. The Bonnie who died was an intelligent, confident, talented girl capable of anything she tried. The Bonnie who lived was lost in the world she came back to. The Bonnie who lived was sure she was dead. I thought a near death experience in intensive care was what left me confused about my existence. It turns out that being unsure of my own existence was just another consequence of severe head trauma.

The first indication of physical problems occurred in college when strange sensations flowed through my body at random moments. An on-campus cardiologist diagnosed hyperventilation and taught me breathing techniques. Starting in college and lasting through my twenties, my menstrual cramps were severe enough for my gynecologist to diagnose that for one day out of each month my body would go into shock. At the time, these seemed like independent, random events, but later I learned about the possibility of hormonal imbalance after traumatic injury, and that these were not random events at all.

They say families of the victims of brain injury think in terms of days or even hours until the victim recovers, but victims themselves think in terms of years. That is certainly true of me. Scholastic difficulty, abusive relationships and severe depression defined the next ten years. All I wanted to do was support myself through college, find a great love, and start a career. It seemed like a simple life plan that everyone around me had no problem achieving. Embarrassed that I struggled ineffectively with these goals, I never told anyone how hard this phase of my life was.

Making good grades in high school had required little or no effort. In college, any class involving memorization was nearly impossible to pass. Defining a scholastic goal was a challenge that kept losing focus. Every time I struggled, I turned against myself, castigating myself as inadequate and stupid.

My relationships with everyone had changed. One day, I read a letter my brother had written to our grandmother. He wrote, "It's like I don't even know Bonnie anymore." My feelings were hurt. At that time, I had no idea brain injury could change personality.

I could not let go of relationships that were long over, and I could not connect with people who offered stable and good relationships. There were beacons of light that I never saw. My grandmother would periodically ask, "Bonnie, are you sure you're all right? You know, you had some really bad injuries." I just dismissed her. When the love of my life asked me to marry him, instead of feeling elation, it felt like he pulled the rug out from under my feet. I knew something was wrong but I could not articulate what.

I wish I had known that the sequelae of traumatic brain injury could include emotional instability, dependent behavior, difficulty with planning and adapting to change and difficulty making decisions based on a lot of simultaneous input. I wish I had known that one of the most common consequences of TBI is depression.

Amnesia allowed me the ability to drive again without fear. Ironically, seeking counseling for a debilitating fear of flying is when I learned that I have post-traumatic stress disorder from the accident. A diagnosis of PTSD finally inspired me to learn the full extent of my injuries and the potential long-term effects. What I learned was enlightening. When I look now at the ramifications of brain trauma, I can see that all of the residual effects were conditions I attributed to my own failures and inadequacy. The evidence that I was still suffering physically from the concussion throughout my twenties, has given me permission to forgive myself for those years. My perspective has changed from regret to wisdom.

Along with the wisdom came clarity. Interestingly, only recently a recurring dream became clear. Over the past several years, in times of high stress, the same dream would repeat all night. In the dream, I was standing over a sink and a nurse was telling me to keep my eyes closed while she washed my hair. I got agitated and told her that she was hurting me and that I wanted my grandmother to wash my hair. The nurse tried to keep me calm by telling me that she was doing the best she could and to keep my eyes closed. "You wouldn't want your grandmother to wash your hair tonight," she said. I opened my eyes anyway and saw a metal sink full of bloody suds. This dream finally stopped occurring when I realized it was not, in fact, a dream, but instead, a memory.

The gaps in my historical memory have fully returned as the healing took place. Eventually, I worked my way through college and graduated summa cum laude. I've been successful in two professions and I have a wonderful network of life-long friends and family that surrounds me. Healing ultimately took counseling, bravery and time, yet I have also found understanding and forgiveness and much more of the Bonnie I once knew.

~Bonnie L. Beuth

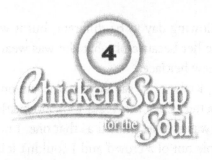

Missing Faces

Caress the detail, the divine detail.
~Vladimir Nabokov

My daughter and I bumped heads while we were roughhousing. The next day, I experienced a severe headache and dizziness and was diagnosed with a moderate concussion. Luckily my daughter came out of it perfectly fine, but for me this concussion was the last in a string of six or more that occurred within a five-year span. The repetitive injuries had a cumulative effect and I ended up with neurologic damage that far surpassed what one would expect from a simple knock on the head by a six-year-old.

I remember very little from my recovery period, but there is one thing that I have never been able to forget. On my first day back at work I went to pick up my daughter at school. As I looked at the group of twenty or so children, I became confused—I did not know which child was mine. I tried to think about the clothes she had on in the morning, but I remembered I had left home before she got up. I felt sick to my stomach and my hands started to sweat as I searched every face.

Thankfully my daughter came forward and said, "Hi Mom." I acted as if nothing was wrong.

I mentioned this incident to no one because it frightened me. Was I losing my mind? Was there more wrong with my brain than I thought? How could a mother not recognize her own daughter? I expected the following day to be different, but it wasn't. I was only able to recognize her because of what she was wearing and her hair, not because I knew her face.

Out of fear, I never did say anything to anyone about it and it never got any better. Over the years I experienced other problems, but no incident was ever as painful as that one. I noticed I had trouble picking people out of a crowd and I couldn't follow movies with lots of different characters in them. I also had trouble at work since I couldn't put names to faces even though I had known my coworkers for many years

Eventually I learned to cope with these problems by using social crutches so people would not know the full extent of my problems. I always asked people what they would be wearing when we were to meet in a crowd or I paid close attention to a person's hairstyle, purse or favorite jewelry to help me recognize them.

If my daughter and I ever went someplace where we might be separated I dressed her in a bright color, usually lime green, so I could find her easily. When she began picking out her own clothes I just made careful note of what she had on before we got out of the car. Once I got a camera phone I often made an excuse to take her picture to have with me in case I lost her in a crowd.

Despite all this, life went on and I just learned to deal with my shortcomings. I never talked about it with anyone. I was too afraid it was a sign of something bigger being wrong and that I was the only one who couldn't recognize her daughter, or her parents or even herself in a mirror.

It wasn't until three years ago that I stumbled upon an Internet article about the rising incidence of prosopagnosia, commonly known as face blindness. As I read, I knew I had found my problem. I finally knew I wasn't crazy. I devoured every word in the article and then searched for more.

I learned that face blindness is a brain disorder where the affected person can't recognize faces the same way a normal person can. The brain functions normally in other ways, but the one area of the brain that controls the memory of faces has been damaged by injury or was malformed during development.

Humans are able to remember many more faces than they can other complex objects due to the way we piece the facial features together and see them as a whole. People with face blindness are unable to do this. They must look at each part of a person's face and use other ways of matching the pieces up to recognize a person. Often a person with face blindness will rely on some other quality such as voice, hairstyle or gait to identify people rather than using facial recognition.

The day I read that article, a great weight was lifted from my shoulders. Finally I had some explanation for the problems I had. I wasn't going crazy and I wasn't alone. Although there is no therapy or treatment for the disorder, I was still left with peace of mind that it was a known problem and finally I could share it with others. It wasn't just me.

These days I am very honest with folks about my inability to recognize people. I tell them straight out that *they* need to find *me* in a crowd and that they shouldn't be upset if I don't recognize them in passing. This is just how I am now. Most people find the condition fascinating and I've run into a couple of people who, upon hearing me mention it, have researched it themselves and have realized that they or a loved one also have the disorder.

You might think that there is nothing good about this story, but you'd be very wrong about that. I consider my face blindness a blessing because it has helped me to live a fuller life.

Before I had that last concussion I was a very shy person who never talked to strangers. I kept to myself and tried to blend into the background. I never went out of my comfort zone and I missed out on many things life has to offer. But now that I don't recognize anyone, I consider everyone a potential new friend! I am more outgoing and eager to talk to people around me and become involved in life.

I've read that some people with face blindness go the other way and become scared to go out and suffer from anxiety and isolation as a result of not recognizing anyone. I can completely understand why that happens, but for me it's been such a positive thing, such a liberating experience. I have so much fun talking to people and learning new things from them now that I can't possibly feel bad about what has happened to me.

Every day is a chance for me to meet someone new and I think that is pretty great.

~Shawn Marie Mann

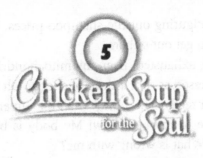

The Land of TBI

To be a hero or a heroine, one must give an order to oneself.

~Simone Weil

It's a Godforsaken place, the land of the brain-injured. The world has changed; it has accelerated to beyond warp speed. With the volume turned up WAY TOO HIGH and the artificial lights, all Broadway spotlights making you cringe and beg for earplugs and sunglasses. The trees swaying with the wind makes you unsteady. In Harvard Square, the sea of people coming and going makes the solid brick sidewalk morph into a floating dock. How can I feel seasick walking on land?

I made it! I'm at the pharmacy, ready to get my medication. I stand in line. My body feels heavier and heavier as I wait for my turn. Finally I give my identification information to the pharmacist who asks if I have any questions. I give him my CVS card, I swipe my debit card. There are so many steps and so much to keep track of. The people are waiting behind me. I am slow. I need to put everything back in the right place in my purse or I will freak out not finding it later.

Finally done with my medication purchase, I pull out my shopping list. Looking at a shelf of shampoo, I am overwhelmed by the infinite choices. And how do I calculate my coupon value? What is best, a dollar off or the 2 for 1 special? Come on brain, it's just math. Simple math. But my brain won't work. Oh how effortlessly she ran before. Oh the glorious before. Stop, don't compare. What am I doing here? Oh, right. Figuring out the shampoo prices. No, I can't do it. Forget it. I have to get out of here.

I'm too tired, exhausted. Even my mitochondria are depleted. I am crashing, no reserves, not a drop of energy. Oh no, I really have to sit down, I feel really sick. I pray to all the Super Heroes, "Please, teleport me home to my bed, now! My body is betraying me left, right and center. What is wrong with me?"

The real kicker is that I look normal. I look like absolutely nothing is wrong with me. Some of my friends don't even believe I'm sick. "You sure do look great," they say. I think to myself, "I am not even a human being anymore."

Patience. So many people tell me to be patient. Why doesn't the pharmaceutical industry encapsulate patience in a little pill? I need really high doses, 24/7. I couldn't tell you how many hours I spend resting, waiting and waiting. Rest. My brain needs lots of rest. I'm generally not a couch potato kinda gal, folks. All this resting, all this waiting to feel better.... my sense of self, my identity is evaporating.

If you are feeling stranded and forlorn in the Land of TBI, try some of these survival tidbits:

Develop a Super Compassionate Self: Sounds dorky but the sooner you excel at this, the easier your life will feel. Super Compassionate Self has special daggers and arrows to take down and destroy toxic opinions, thoughts and attitudes from within and a special shield for external toxicity. Super Compassionate Self is always on the lookout for anything that will make you smile, laugh or feel better. SCS makes the time for relaxation, pleasure and enjoyment because these are mandatory to help offset the poisons in the Land of TBI.

Energy Voids: This is a normal weather pattern in TBI Land. Don't take the weather personally. On "extremely nasty bad flu with a really mean hangover" days, just stay in bed, take your healing tablets, drink soothing beverages, and be mellow. These are refueling days and if you don't take them, you will hit the Wall. Unavoidably you will be forced to hit the Wall. You cannot hide in your flurry of errands or cleaning or working or whatever you seem to think you must do. Denying that the Wall WILL find you, will often make you hit it harder. You are NOT rewarded in TBI Land for going beyond your limits. You are actually penalized. You will have ugly consequences like migraines, nausea, vomiting, prolonged fatigue lasting longer than you could think possible for a living person. You may have severe anxiety attacks or feel tremendous despair. Like the Dementors in *Harry Potter*, these emotions can suck the life out of your soul.

Antidotes: Hoard excellent Nurturing Catalysts. Fresh flowers near your bed or resting spots, peaceful music or nature sounds, soothing smells like lavender candles or favorite teas. Regular massage or citrus lotion to rub into your hands and feet. Nurturing Catalysts are more powerful than they appear and they have tremendous synergistic capabilities. DEFINITELY the more the merrier! Laughter, truckloads of laughter or clouds of laughter, get regular doses.

Paradox Reigns: Awareness that life is much more complicated and much more simple at the same time. Many priorities will change drastically, many people will never understand, you have things to be grateful for. You will love more deeply and curse more emphatically and your favorite ice cream will taste even sweeter. It is wise to become as flexible as possible with your concepts of everything. What used to be fun can now feel like very hard work. What used to be work could be something you wish desperately you could do. Taking a shower can some days feel like a huge task. A cup of tea can feel like a friend. Sunshine on your face, like a vacation.

A new life 101: Study and learn the intricacies of your limitations, live as much as possible in this zone for optimal energy efficiency. Be outrageously impressed with all that you have experienced in the Land of TBI. You are way more advanced than any *Candy Crusher*. You are one tough cookie. Not as a video character, IN REAL LIFE. You are your own hero.

Bask in your exquisiteness and the genuine glory of YOU. Just the way you are. Yup, just exactly the way you are. Right now. You "be" amaaaaZING!

~Catz LeBlanc

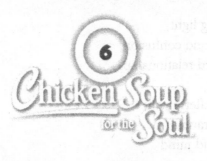

Mirror, Mirror

We convince by our presence.
~Walt Whitman

Anger, sadness, confusion
are there
on the face
of the one

watching,
learning,
mirroring.

Crow's feet wrinkled.
Corners crinkled.
Gray hair hide-and-seek.
How long the age clues?

I closed my eyes and willed the memories
To anchor the present
To the realities.

Once I wanted it to be over.
All of it:

The pain,

the blinding light,
arguments and confusion,
and wrecked relationships.

So much suffering after
the initial trauma.
My body and mind
held hostage
in rips, tears and scars.

Curiosity stepped in…
What did I know?
What didn't I remember?
Would I ever recover?
… to save me.

I touch my face,
then my cool reflection.
Thankful that
How, What, When, and Who
are no longer
as important as

I am.

~Donna Stamey Reeve

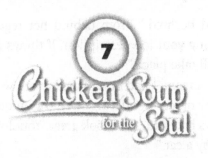

Invisible Bruise

Better to light a candle than to curse the darkness.
~Chinese Proverb

I walked past the cracked-open door of the conference room, and overheard the health department director speaking to my supervisor. "Melissa needs to be fired." I ran back to my cubby, trembling, and shuffled protocols from one pile to another without purpose. I paused at one that needed revising, but the algorithm of circles and squares looked like Rorschach inkblots.

Maybe the director had heard about my misunderstanding with a coworker a few weeks earlier: "The protocol isn't ready to be submitted. I told you it needs another revision." Maybe my supervisor had told the director about my experience at the pediatric clinic. The brightly-lit windowless rooms and wailing infants had made me dizzy. By the end of day one, my head felt as if it had been filled with jelly and my body like it was stuffed into a box. At the time, my supervisor had agreed that it was not the place for me. "I think you'll do better working on specific projects." Did she know something I didn't?

Despite the threat of being fired, I continued to go to work. During meetings, the other nurses spoke too fast and their voices sounded distant, as if they weren't in the room with me. I had never felt disconnected from my peers before. My eyes twitched with fatigue, and I jotted notes just to keep myself awake. But the notes quickly turned into stars and moons and crosshatched lines.

After two weeks of little sleep, I confronted the director. "I heard you say I should be fired." From behind her regal desk, she said, "You're not fulfilling your job description. If things don't change, the firing process will take place."

I wanted to scream. I had never failed in the workplace before. I walked out of her office, wondering what was wrong with me. After all, my coworkers had said, "You look great. You don't even look like you've been hit by a car."

Rather than be fired, I searched for another job, and accepted a part-time position at a pediatrician's office. "It's been a long time since you've worked in a clinical setting," the doctor said. "Do you think you're capable?"

"Oh yes," I said, with false confidence. For two weeks, I watched a veteran nurse measure patients' heights and weights, then plot them on graphs. I watched her prick babies' heels for blood samples. I can do this, I thought. I've done this before. She administered vaccines to toddlers, pinning them down as they kicked and screamed and spit. My ears rang and my heart thumped behind my ribs.

I misread vaccine labels and administered the wrong one to a toddler. I misread measurements, and when I plotted them on patients' graphs, my dots fell far below or far above the others. There were too many dots, like a pointillism painting. I hoped no one would notice my mistakes, so I didn't tell anyone. I answered calls from parents, but fell behind in the conversation, because I couldn't scribble notes fast enough. When I looked back at them, they made no sense: is that an M or an N? A three or an eight? Coworkers often said, "Can you explain what this means?"

"How do you think things are going?" my supervisor asked during my first review two months later.

"Pretty good," I ventured.

She then listed my failings: inaccurate patient measurements, insufficient blood samples, too much time assessing patients. I agreed to a one-month probation. The month passed. "Melissa, your ability to keep pace is still concerning," she said. "Do you think this job is a good fit for you?"

"I enjoy working with kids," I stuttered.

She offered another two weeks probation. That same day, I had to re-administer an eye exam to a three-year-old, because the first time I had used flashcards designed for older children. During the next review, the pediatrician met with me. "Parents are dissatisfied with your injection techniques," he said, slapping his palm against the desk. "Calls aren't being returned, and you continually use the wrong forms to document babies' feeding history." Another slap. "Have you had problems in the workplace before?"

"No, never." I didn't want to tell him about the health department.

When he offered me another chance, with reduced work responsibilities, and pay, I said I'd think about it—I was ashamed to accept the pay cut. The next day, I scheduled an appointment for neuropsychological testing to assess the reason for my difficulties in the workplace.

I spent an entire day in the neuropsychologist's office, where he tested my attention span, memory, language skills, and executive function—the ability to engage in complex thinking. He showed me a photograph and asked me to name it. I twisted my lips, chewed on them. The word was so close.

"Sph," he hinted.

"Sphinx!" I yelled.

He asked me to draw a simple diagram from memory, but the pencil tip grated against the page, making random lines and obtuse angles. Then he asked me to recite words beginning with the letter T. "Top, tired, toy, trumpet..."

"Time's up," he said, and clicked the stopwatch.

A few weeks later, I received the report in the mail:

"Melissa's cognitive functioning is guarded, as it has been three years since her injury and research suggests that most cognitive recovery following a traumatic brain injury takes place during the first two years. Mild recovery could occur if she engages in cognitive rehabilitation."

I crumpled the report into a ball and threw it across the room. I caught a whiff of the roses on the dining room table, and realized I was actually relieved. I un-crumpled the report. Finally, I knew why

I moved slowly, why bright lights made me dizzy, why I misread vaccine labels.

The neuropsychologist referred me to a cognitive therapist. She explained that the parts of the brain cells called axons were likely damaged, resulting in a disruption in communication between neurons: the reason for my unusual fatigue and difficulty with multitasking and concentration. She encouraged me to pace myself and keep an activity schedule, even for things like brushing my teeth, which I regularly forgot to do until the afternoon. She introduced me to the name game where you repeat a person's name back to them when first introduced: "Hi Margaret. It's nice to meet you, Margaret." She taught me a method for evoking images to recall things like groceries: balancing my feet on a gallon of milk or putting a pound of green beans on my head.

It took me years to train and accept my rewired brain. Living with a traumatic brain injury connected me with professionals who offered hope, ways to cope with multiple stimuli, whether at a party or in the grocery store. They reminded me that TBIs are often not visible. Now, a decade later, people still say, "You look great. You don't even look like you've been hit by a car." I twist my lips, trying to find the right words. Finally, with a smile, I say, "Thank you. You don't either."

~Melissa Cronin

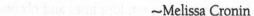

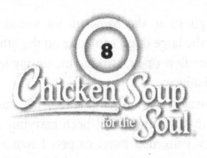

Learning to Live with a Label

A sudden bold and unexpected question doth many times
surprise a man and lay him open.

~Francis Bacon

I'd waited only a few minutes when the doctor stepped into the room. She was as short as me, with large round glasses and thick wavy brown hair held back by the kind of clip my daughter would wear. She looked young, but I knew she had earned her place in the neurology department of the University of Colorado hospital through years of study and practice.

I watched as she picked up a manila folder and began to scan its contents. I read the label on the file and began to feel irritated. "Why is she reviewing another patient's chart during my appointment?" I wondered. "Maybe the charts are switched and she doesn't know she's reading the wrong one."

"Excuse me," I interrupted. "I think you have the wrong file." She glanced up at me, then at the file, "No, this is your file," she said. I protested, "But that label says 'epilepsy', and I don't have epilepsy." She closed the folder and scooted closer.

"You are Joy, right?" she began gently, pointing to my name. "And some years ago, you suffered a traumatic brain injury, right?" Yes. She was right. In the spring of 1996, I had been the program director for the annual Youth for Christ staff conference. Early one morning,

I was escorting guests to the ballroom for sound checks and, as I reached to open the large door, someone on the other side leaned on it. The heavy door flew open, striking me on my left temple, knocking me into the hallway.

I was unconscious for only a few seconds, and when I opened my eyes, I saw that the things I'd been carrying were now strewn across the boldly patterned hotel carpet. I remember thinking, "I need to pick those up. I need to get back to work." But I was unable to move or speak.

Several friends hovered over me, their eyes betraying their concern. My first words assured them, "I'm okay." But after a few questions resulting in the same answer, a wise friend asked a question to which my response of "I'm okay" proved that I was certainly not okay.

A few minutes later, I sat up and tried to talk, but was stuttering. I had a nasty headache, but when people around me asked if I wanted them to call an ambulance, I shrugged it off. "It was just a bump on the head," I thought, as my pride overrode my better judgment.

I was too proud to admit that a "little" bump on the head could get in my way. I was also too proud of my work to step aside, letting other competent people take over. The program could certainly have gone on without me if I'd been wise enough to let it go while I went to the hospital.

Looking back, I now know those voices in my head weren't healthy responses. And today, everyone involved would know better than to believe a person who has just been smacked in the head when she says, "I'm okay." But in the mid 1990's, everyone was still learning how to recognize and treat traumatic brain injuries.

When I returned to my home in Denver after the accident, I made an appointment with a neurologist who ordered many tests. She saw the contusion on my brain and prescribed appropriate treatments. I had medications for the excruciating migraines, I learned compensation strategies in occupational therapy, and I began speech therapy for the aphasia.

That was a new word for me: aphasia, literally translated, "nonspeaking." I had been an English major in college; I liked to write and I enjoyed speaking at conferences. So struggling with words was a new experience for me. Words had been my friends: creative words, expressive words, accurate words, many words! But because of the brain injury, words failed me.

Even after I recovered from stuttering, I struggled to find the correct words to fit a situation. I could think accurately about a concept, but I couldn't speak the right word. I recall watching an injured bird in our back yard and saying to my husband, "How is that poor bird ever going to swim out of here?"

The doctor who treated me in 1996 was one of Denver's best neurologists. She prescribed good methods for recovery and convinced me to wait another year to attend graduate school. She warned me, "When you do go to school, don't expect great academic ability. Your brain injury will interfere with learning languages, and you will struggle with remembering dates and other details." Eighteen months after the accident, I followed my inner calling and enrolled in the Denver Seminary where I would need to learn Greek and Hebrew and remember many dates and details.

I soon began to notice that every now and then, my mind went blank. These blanks were never long or severe, so I wasn't especially concerned. Thinking I was cured from my brain injury, I assumed these blips were just part of normal aging and I never told a doctor about them.

I loved seminary! I stretched the coursework out over seven years, working in several churches and adopting two daughters during that time. Finally, in May of 2004, I stood on the platform graduating with my classmates. At our celebration party, a friend reminded me what the neurologist had said eight years earlier about lowering my expectations. Apparently, I had not followed those instructions very well because I graduated as the valedictorian and, in a stunning surprise, I also earned that year's preaching award.

But my failure to deal with those little blank moments was about to catch up with me. Nine months after graduation, following complications for an unrelated surgery, my brain finally cried out for the attention it needed. I slipped into an extended absence or petit mal seizure and was rushed to the hospital. A week of intensive care and research into my history of head injury resulted in a more accurate word for those momentary blips in consciousness: micro-seizures.

I was referred to the neurology department at the university where, a year later, my new doctor walked into my life and told me the truth: that my brain injury had caused a condition that fell on the epilepsy spectrum. It's just a label, but it is an ominous word. I'll never know why no previous doctor told me about the label, or why I never figured it out in my own research. I've wondered to myself what would have happened if I had known about the label earlier. Would I have excused myself from working hard or might I have avoided trying things that were out of my comfort zone? Would I have limited myself by wearing the epileptic label?

Looking back, I'm thankful for the time that I didn't know about the label on my file. I might have missed out on great opportunities. I'm also thankful that the doctor told me the truth at a time when I was ready to face my label, but not wear it.

~Joy Engelsman

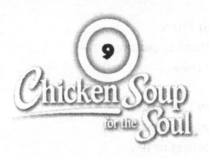

Who Am I?

Not until we are lost do we begin to understand ourselves.
~Henry David Thoreau

There was a time
When I was not like this
But now the tables have turned

And now I am not sure
Who I am
Or what I have become

Especially since now
I am not who I used to be

Communication breakdown
Can't seem to find the words
Or understand when spoken to

Anger—Confusion—Frustration—Depression
It's sometimes a desperate and overwhelming situation

Feeling lost in so much confusion
And losing my confidence
In what I say or do

And although I have
A natural instinct to survive
Just hear my cries

For right now I just need
Friendship and understanding
Not false promises or lies

So please don't walk out
And slam the door on me

For the memories of my past
Will always remind me
Of who I once used to be

But I have the ambition and drive
And I will find the means to survive

For I will be
Who I want to be

~Donna Fitzpatrick

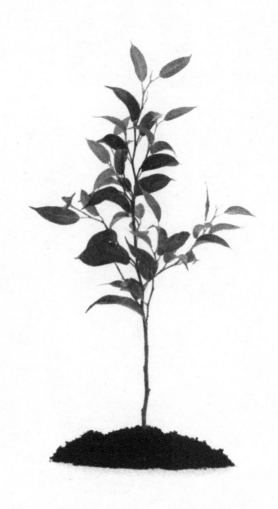

Chapter
2

Recovering *from* Traumatic Brain Injuries

Self-Discovery

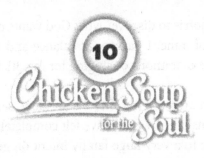

Treasures from Tragedy

Example is leadership.
~Albert Schweitzer

I t is difficult to find treasures in the midst of a devastating tragedy, but there is always beauty to be found among the ashes.

It was spring 1997. I was enjoying my new little family in Little Rock, Arkansas. I had married and moved five hundred miles away from my family and friends in Louisville, Kentucky two years before. I saw it as an adventure! I was starting a new life in a new town with a new husband… and now a precious baby, Andrew.

As I was driving to a cookout with my three-month-old son in tow, my happy life changed in an instant when my car was t-boned by a teenager on a neighborhood street. An emergency room nurse witnessed my collision. That was the first of many blessings, as he ran over and administered CPR to get me breathing again. The second blessing was that Andrew was unharmed, asleep in his car seat. God saved our lives that day. That was the ultimate blessing.

I have no memory of my accident or the months I spent in the hospital. After being comatose for two months, I graduated from critical care to the brain injury unit. My family members in Louisville kept tabs on me through my parents, who rented an apartment in Little Rock during my hospital stay. They still like to tell funny stories about my behavior during that time. That is one of the treasures of having a brain injury. I can't remember the awful and inappropriate things I said and did during my immediate recovery.

My current job is to discover what God wants me to do with this interrupted life of mine. I have poor balance and an odd sounding voice, so no more marathons or singing for me. It's time to develop a new set of skills!

My husband divorced me after the accident, sending me back to my family in Louisville. I would have felt completely abandoned had I not come home to a very large family intent on getting me back to a high-functioning and happy life. I'm heartbroken to have missed my son's childhood. Life has not turned out as I dreamed, but I could not have been the best parent and also continued the hard work of rebuilding myself. My son was well cared for in my absence and is a fine young man today. Another treasure!

I can still remember that evening when my father and I arrived home in Louisville from packing my belongings in Little Rock. One by one, family members came over to welcome me home. My sister Julie helped me unpack and organize my clothes. It was a loving gesture. But since we are the same size, I think she might have been looking for things to borrow, too.

My family's desire to help me led them to the Brain Injury Alliance of Kentucky (BIAK) that serves brain injury survivors and the families who care for them. My brothers Dan and Andrew, my sister-in-law Ann, and I have all spent time serving on their board of directors. The real treasure that came from all of this was that my family began and organized the first Brain Ball in 2004, a gala that raises money to enable BIAK to continue helping and supporting the brain injury community. I have the privilege of choosing another brain injury survivor each year to receive the award, honoring their courage, perseverance and service to others. The Brain Ball has become one of the most prestigious fundraisers in Louisville. And it always leaves my family feeling grateful that they began this wonderful affair.

But since the Brain Ball happens just once a year, what could I do to make my life useful the other 364 days? With no family to care for anymore, what was my purpose? Before the accident, I would go for long runs to ponder such questions. Now I go for long, slow walks. I have always been very regimented and dedicated to getting enough exercise to stay healthy and fit. Could I make something useful for others out of my passion for fitness?

Intent on finding a new purpose, I began studying and ultimately became a certified personal trainer. A therapist from Vocational Rehab suggested I teach exercise classes in senior homes and facilities. They even purchased a portable sound system and microphone so that students could hear my soft voice over the music I play. In 2010, my career in Senior Fitness was launched!

My classes are relaxed and fun. Students sit in, or stand by, a chair while stretching and toning their muscles. My years as a physical therapy patient have given me much insight into how the muscles work together to produce a strong and flexible body. All the balance training I have received has given me even more tips and cues to share with my class. Balance work is important for everyone as they age.

My local newspaper featured a story about the classes I teach. It recognized some of the seniors in the class and celebrated how they were able to become stronger, while having a good time in the process. My classes were so well received that I went back to study for another certification as a Senior Fitness Instructor. A friend in the marketing and advertising business designed a logo and webpage for my business, Silver Strength.

My disability seems to bring out the good in people. It certainly brought out the kindness and generosity in my four brothers. Since my brain injury, I can no longer drive. I have a driver to get me to and from classes on time. Since I pay my drivers more than I charge for a class, I must teach two classes each day to have my income exceed my expenses. My brothers cover my driver expense, allowing me to enjoy my little income.

Another treasure is that a family friend started a scholarship at my high school for a student exhibiting courage and determination under hard circumstances. It's called the Mary Varga Life of Courage award. It's such a thrill for me to see the scholarship recipient's excitement and gratitude when his or her name is called. I was also selected for membership in my high school's Hall of Fame. It was such an honor and a testament to how far I have been able to go since I graduated from Assumption High School.

All of these blessings and treasures have not taken away my disabilities or the difficulty they add to my life. But these treasures show me that if you keep trying and laughing and loving, in spite of your problems, others will be inspired to make an impact in their own little corner of the world.

~Mary Varga

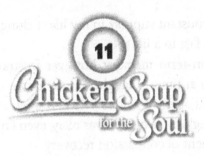

Lights... Camera... Action!

No one remains quite what he was when he recognizes himself.

~Thomas Mann

It was as if someone else were performing the role of me. This woman acted like me, yet I did not know her. "She wore that?" I asked when I opened her closet and looked through her clothes. "She ate that?" when I peeked in the fridge and pantry. How odd, this former self was.

As the months passed, as the seasons changed, I struggled with the new me. The reflection in the mirror wasn't me—or was it? I gradually accepted that the image I viewed was me. I experienced a reluctant reawakening of the senses. Who am I? What am I like? Will I return to who I was before the accident? Did I want to? Did I have to? Endless questions came and went unanswered.

Comments from the public were often heartless or at least unthinking. The cashiers were impatient in response to the confusion caused by my concussion. I didn't know how to hand over the correct amount of cash. Shopping for groceries was difficult as there were too many choices and overwhelming sensory stimulation. Do I buy one or two cans? Do I like bananas? A concussion cannot be seen from the outside, only experienced from within. The people around me did not understand my journey through concussion recovery.

One day, the concussion fog lifted ever so slightly and a glimpse of my new self emerged. Slowly I felt more awake, more alive. It was a gradual return from the depths of darkness. My sons and their families were a constant support in my life. I clung to this lifeline, as a survivor holds fast to a life raft.

Loss of short-term memory, however frustrating, was actually somewhat funny at times. I laughed at my errant comments. Seeing the reaction on people's faces was priceless when my response was a little offbeat. Laughing at myself was okay, even encouraged. Humor is a healing element of concussion recovery.

I slowly returned to my job. It was not easy, but then the important things in life never are. Part of what made my return to work so difficult is that it was in the very act of doing my job—delivering mail as an office services worker for a local oil company—that I suffered my TBI. But a steady voice in my head urged me forward even though sometimes I progressed backwards. My doctor assured me that setbacks were a normal part of recovery, so I pushed on. I slowly, reluctantly accepted my new self, discovered new skills and mourned the loss of old ones.

Lights... Camera... Action! My new life rolled by scene after scene. The credits rolled too, paying tribute to the actor who played my life over the past year. I am that actor. I am a survivor and I love the new me!

~Sandra L. Brown

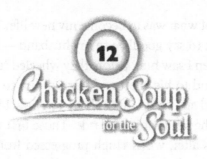

Flashes of Hope

Truth is the torch that gleams through the fog without dispelling it.
~Claude Adrien Helevetius

The lights were down low as Hugh and I watched the movie *Vanilla Sky* on television while our twin daughters were out at a middle school dance. When I rented the movie, I knew nothing about it; I was in a hurry and liked the title. Near the beginning of the film, a jealous girlfriend takes her cheating lover on a wild car ride, intent on killing them both in a crash. My muscles tensed as the car veered out of control and flew over a bridge. I wanted to turn the movie off, but I couldn't. I sat frozen, my heart racing. Hugh sat in the recliner next to me. When I glanced over at him, his face looked blank, like he might doze off. He's always in a trance, I thought. The movie continued, disorienting me with its emotionally violent twists and turns.

Only two months before, Hugh had left the house for an afternoon workout on his bicycle. He was a seasoned athlete who had completed many bike races and triathlons. I had dropped off our daughters at a local skating rink for the afternoon, picked up some groceries and driven home. I heard the phone ringing as I unlocked the front door. I set down my paper bags, answered the phone, and heard a frenzied voice say, ""Do you know a cyclist?"

Hugh had been struck by a car and rushed to MCV Hospital in Richmond, Virginia. When I arrived at the emergency room, a policewoman, trauma coordinator, and chaplain tried to guide me through the initial hour of what was to become my new life. The chaplain told me I might want to say goodbye to my husband—he had a massive head injury. When I saw him, before they wheeled him up for surgery, I pressed my hand to his chest and begged him to hold on. He was unconscious, and all I could think about was how I hadn't kissed him goodbye before he left for his bike ride. Those first moments and the thirty-three days after, when Hugh progressed from the ICU to the step-down unit to the acute brain injury rehabilitation center, felt like a bad dream that slowly morphed me into a vague, foggy replica of my former self.

When Hugh woke up from his coma, his eyes looked dazed and empty, as if his soul had left his body. Slowly, he began to move, walk, and speak, though his speech was raspy and irregular. In my bed alone at night, I wondered: Did my husband die in that accident?

The surgeon removed a large chunk of Hugh's skull and put it in the hospital freezer until his brain swelling receded. He said it would take about three months before they would put him back together. In the meantime, I was told to keep a close eye on him. Hugh was sent home with a canvas gait belt around his waist that I would hold to keep him upright, and a thick white helmet to protect his skull. I signed papers as his designated "guardian."

At home, Hugh alternated between agitation, sitting in his recliner dismantling the remote, and falling asleep from the exhaustion brought on by short bouts of rehab. He was nothing like his former self, so I don't know why I glanced over at him as if he could shield me from the violence of the movie I was watching, but our eyes met, and for a second, I thought he actually saw me. A little while later, my cell phone rang during an intense movie sequence, and I jumped before answering it.

"Hi, hon. I'm thinking of you." Hugh's whispery voice said.

I glanced over at him, sitting nearby in his recliner. His eyes softened in an old familiar way, a way that I had not seen since before the accident. He was holding his cell phone and staring straight at me. My mind, still confused from the dream sequence of the movie, felt tricked again. Was Hugh really calling me now? Had I fallen asleep? Did his eyes really crease in that old way of his? I played along. Slowly I rose from the couch and walked away from him into the dining room, holding my cell phone tight like a lifeline.

"I'm right here. Don't you like the movie?" I asked.

"It's okay," he said.

"Why did you call me? We're in the same room."

"I was just thinking about you so I thought I'd call and tell you."

"That is very sweet. Are you courting me?"

"I guess," he said. I held my phone through long silences as we talked for a while longer. We talked more that night than we usually did over a full day. I was transported back in time as I stood in my dining room, speaking to my husband only steps away. For the rest of the evening, we watched each other more than the movie. I kept staring at him, amazed that he was alive. He kept staring at me as if trying to get to know me all over again.

In the movie, an eerie voice says, "Open your eyes." The main character's conscience plays tricks on him. He's in a coma, and he's battling inner demons of vanity, love, and righting past wrongs. He's lost, confused, struggling, and hiding. That night, alone with my husband in the house, I fell in love again with the past and present version of my husband.

These momentary flashes of my pre-accident husband were flashes of hope, a fulfillment of longing. After that night, I would seek them out, and notice each familiar character trait returned to me like a gift as his brain slowly healed. The months and years passed, and somewhere along the way, the fog lifted, and there stood my husband, not my old husband, or my new husband, just my husband as he was simply meant to be.

~Rosemary Rawlins

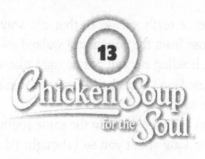

Man of the House

Think positively about yourself…. ask God who made you
to keep on remaking you.

~Norman Vincent Peale

"I'm in a New York state of mind," were the lyrics ringing out so joyfully from the Billy Joel song on the radio. They put a smile on my face that lingered throughout the entire song.

It was a Friday evening in January and I didn't personally know about that New York state of mind, but I was definitely in a "TGIF" state of mind. For some reason, it seemed like the past week had been the longest I had ever worked. It had felt like Friday would never come.

As I approached the highway ramp to get onto the expressway, my mind lingered for a moment on a nice hot bath and some good old-fashioned chicken soup to warm my tired aching body.

I turned the radio up to hear some more sweet music to make the long ride home more pleasant, but the music stopped and an announcement came on the radio that there had been an accident on the expressway. A car turned over and drivers were using just one lane. I turned away from the entrance ramp and headed down a side street, thinking that it would probably extend my journey home by at least another hour and a half. My hot bath was looking more like a quick shower and the good old hot chicken soup was looking more like a cold turkey sandwich.

Although the route I decided to take was the longest route home,

I would avoid the traffic. I smiled like some conquering hero, figuring that I had handled that situation pretty well.

As I drove, the lights were all green. However, as I entered an intersection, I noticed an SUV waiting in the turn lane. Having the light still in my favor, I proceeded into the intersection. I was midway across the street when, for some unknown reason, the driver took off and turned in front of my car. I raised my foot to apply the brake and that was the last thing I remember.

While lying in a state of oblivion, I recall that I felt a peace that was beyond comprehension. A progressive feeling of unrestricted freedom surrounded me in complete and total bliss. I was calm and in a fog, and I thought, "I must be dead; if this is heaven, I'm loving it."

All of a sudden, reality set in. I tasted blood and, for the first time, felt pain. Opening my eyes, I realized the Lord had spared my life. He was not through with me yet and there was more that He had for me to do in this life.

The next thing I remember was being cut out of my car and the seatbelt. While they were cutting me loose, I remember calling my wife and telling her that I was involved in a bad accident. They brought the stretcher and strapped me down, put me in the EMS truck, and we headed for the hospital. When I got there, my wife and daughter told me that I had been thrown into the rearview mirror and cut my head. I also had seatbelt burns across my chest, two sprained wrists, and lacerations on my legs.

I stayed in the hospital overnight and had multiple tests. Since my head hit the mirror, they thought I had fractured my neck. The next day I was sent home with orders to see my family physician. But the next morning, when I tried to get out of bed, the entire room started to spin. My wife rushed me back to the hospital, and they told me that I had vertigo. It was so bad that I could not stand without a cane or something to lean on. My equilibrium was completely off and there was not too much they could do for me until my brain healed.

My doctor ordered me to see a psychotherapist, because my attitude and behavior were drastically changing. I was getting irritable with everything and everyone. It was not like me. I had been very quiet and laid back, with most things never moving me out of my comfort zone or getting on my nerves. I had lost my short-term memory and was extremely short-tempered with all my therapists. I did not trust any of them.

What made this behavior so peculiar was that I did not realize the change in myself. At first, I thought that it was just my age catching up with me. But my forgetting had become a constant thing, and I found that I just could not help myself. Even tying strings around my finger to remember to pick up the laundry didn't help. I forgot why I had tied the string around my finger for in the first place. It was the most frightening time of my life.

There were some moments that I did not tell anyone about, because it was too embarrassing. It was so distressing to call home and say that I forgot which street to take to get home. Not only did I forget many streets, but I would get confused about which direction I was going. I would have to pull over on the soft shoulder of the expressway and sit there for a moment to figure out which way the sun was setting in order to get my bearings and figure out which direction I needed to travel.

Being the only man around three women in the house, I felt I needed to protect my manhood. Also they always wanted me to drive when we went out. I felt that it was too demeaning to admit, but deep down inside, I also knew that it was about my stupid pride. I could not help myself. I just wanted to keep that strong protective image that I had with my girls. I did not want to lose that role. But truth be told, I needed them much more than they needed me.

I now have much greater sympathy for those who struggle with Alzheimer's disease and other dementias—the confusion, the secret shame, the pride and sense of purpose that can disappear. I knew that I would get better, but their condition progressively deteriorates. Although I did eventually recover, I will always remember what it feels like to have an injured brain.

~Marshall Campbell

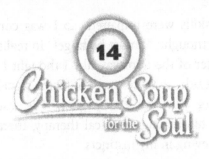

14

Starting Over

If there is one thing that can be forecast with confidence, it is that the future will turn out in unexpected ways.

~Peter F. Drucker

My life changed in a moment. While returning from taking my son and his friend to school, a car crashed into my SUV, causing it to roll. It took the Jaws of Life to remove me from the vehicle, and I remember nothing.

When I woke up in the hospital, I didn't know who I was. I didn't recognize my son or have any knowledge of current events. Who was the President? It was more like what is a President?

I had suffered a traumatic brain injury, which left me with retrograde and anterograde amnesia. My past was totally gone. Doctors told me that my condition was the best it would ever be. A therapist later told me to think of it as if I were a newborn, learning everything from scratch.

Life didn't get easier after being released from the hospital. Day-to-day activities were confusing. Basics like dirty dishes going in the dishwasher and clothes being inside the closet were new concepts. Meanwhile, I had my youngest child, a thirteen-year-old son, to raise. I was trying to learn the duties required of a mother in addition to the basics of functioning at home and in society, and it felt overwhelming. One day, I burned cookies when the kitchen timer in my pocket went off... while I was standing in line at the post office. But give up? Never!

My motor skills were impaired, so I was constantly running into doorways. I thought, "I must be huge!" In reality, I wasn't going through the center of the doorway like I thought I was. I had little feeling on my left side, so there were confusing signals from my brain to my body parts. Pain was ever-present. The rest of my life will always include chiropractic, physical therapy, therapeutic massage, doctors, and believing in my instincts.

Prior to the accident, I ran my own consulting firm specializing in accounting and database management. Returning to consulting was not an option; I would have no idea how to help my clients. In fact, trying to relearn even simple math was a challenge because I couldn't remember the number four—a common problem with my type of brain injury.

I began volunteering for my local hospital's auxiliary, editing the newsletter and raising money. Volunteering helped me learn what functions I was good at and which activities I wasn't able to do.

Friends encouraged me to enroll at Claremont Graduate University, where I earned a certificate in leadership. After lots of hard work, and with the help of patient professors and student-led study groups, I earned my master's degree in management with honors. While at the university, I became a student of Peter F. Drucker, the prominent author and educator. I was fortunate to become friends with him and his wife Doris. They encouraged and inspired me.

While earning my master's degree, I became director of the MBA program at the Peter F. Drucker School of Management. I found my rhythm as a productive, effective team member—bringing alumni, staff, students, and Professor Drucker together for the enrichment of all.

At some point during my journey, I decided to sculpt a personality for myself because I couldn't remember my character traits from before the accident. Based on observing others, I realized that if I became known as a happy person, people would want to be around me. From then on, becoming happy in spite of my circumstances was my mission. It became what I call my "happiness project."

As I focused on being happy, the key was to not dwell on the negative aspects of my life. For example, I made a conscious decision not to lament the absence of special memories, like giving birth to my children. Instead, I concentrated on the present.

I also became determined not to let setbacks destroy my happiness. When I was involved in a second car crash, I suffered another brain injury. It happened as I was finishing my master's degree, and schoolwork was much harder after this second injury. But I decided that happiness is a choice, and I just needed to make a conscious effort to stay positive.

In recent years, I have become focused on speaking, writing, and coaching, to empower people to break through self-imposed barriers, implement new strategies, and achieve successful outcomes, just as I have. I have founded a non-profit organization (www.tbibridge.org) that provides resources for survivors of traumatic brain injury and post-traumatic stress disorder. My motto is "Believe. Be patient. Never give up!"

My life now is rich with close friends, family, and activities I enjoy, in addition to my non-profit work. I don't know what my life was like before the accident, but all that matters is that I'm happy now. Attitude truly is everything!

~Celeste Palmer

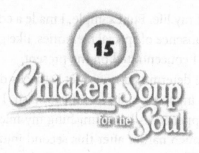

15

My Second Life

Only by joy and sorrow does a person know anything about themselves and their destiny.

~Johann Wolfgang von Goethe

On September 8, 2008, I fell off a building on my former college campus, and I lay dying for more than six hours. Blood was filling my lungs, and I was hardly breathing. At seven the following morning, a maintenance man found me and called for help. They had to resuscitate me, and after they did, I was in a coma for more than a week.

That was how I ended a three-decade-long drug and alcohol habit. It took me thirty years to fall ten feet. When I surfaced from my coma, I was told I had suffered a traumatic brain injury. The only thing I could think of was a cigarette.

"Hey, you got a cigarette?" I asked.

"No," a nurse said, leaving the room, letting me sit with the beeps of the machines.

I had absolutely no idea what was going on, or how badly I was injured. I didn't know that even if the nurse had thrown me an entire pack of cigarettes, I would not have been able to go out and have one, because I could not walk on my own.

After two weeks I left the ICU and transferred to an acute care floor. They said, because of my age, I needed intense therapy. While I was in acute care, I realized what true human beings are, and I came to realize that I was not one of them. I was a fool. During this time, my family and the hospital staff would say, "Well, I hope this is it for you. I hope you change."

One night I again asked a nurse, "You got a cigarette?"

"No."

I fell back on my pillow, and I thought about how many times I had tried to quit this life: the drugs, the liquor, the cigarettes. How many times had people heard me say I was going to quit? Not even my near death could convince them I was serious.

I sat up, and said out loud, "I'm going to change!"

When I put my head down that night, I turned away from all the nonsense that led me to fall. I could do nothing about the past, but I could change every step from here on out. It was the birth of what I consider my second life. I believed then, as I do now, that I have had two lifetimes in one over-all existence.

This second life would be built on the integrity of my actions, so every day I gave the therapist my best, and I gave myself my best. It was all I could do.

The fall on my head left me seeing double, but I had not realized it until a morning shower. My face was paralyzed on the right side, so I resembled a stroke victim. I had broken my right scapula and my right wrist. I had a scar along my ribs where a tube was put in to suck the blood out of my lung. I was in a wheelchair, unable to walk.

After about a month in acute care, I was transferred to the sub-acute floor. It would be there that I would question my entire existence as a human being. Everyone I met in sub-acute care, from patients to staff, had an immense influence on the development of who I would become, who I have become.

Every day I pushed myself both physically and emotionally. I worked hard at all my therapy sessions, did more of each therapy on my own time, and spent the bulk of my off-time in the office of my rehab specialist.

A rehab specialist is like a caseworker. It was in her office that I did an intense investigation of myself. I questioned every belief. I went above and beyond my daily therapy. During these five months,

I began to reshape my belief system. I made a promise to myself, and the "new" Paul kept his promises.

The day I left sub-acute care was a sad day for me. I loved everyone there; they were my family. We would be together forever though, for my heart would carry them the rest of my life.

My work was far from done, because I had no life to get back to, so I had to build one. I sought help, and I realized that I had some emotional problems. In fact, I was an emotional nightmare. I read books about emotion.

I was quick to anger but didn't know what to do when I got angry, until one day, when I was angry; I sat down on the floor and again talked to myself: "This is your anger, Paul, yours to deal with. No one can help you; you have to help yourself."

The only way I could look at the anger was to write about it. When I wrote about it, I could see it, relive what I was angry about, and use that energy for a more productive outcome. With words, I saw who I was. I fell in love with words. I wrote a book about what happened to me; it took me a year.

After that year, I took a class on creative writing; I learned from other writers, and became a writer. It is my destiny, the reason I am here, and the reason I survived near death. I never question that. My TBI taught me the truth of my existence.

~Paul Ceretto

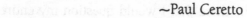

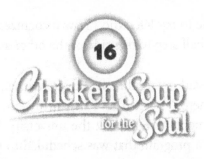

16

Chicken Soup for the Soul

Road to a New Path

Music is a higher revelation than all wisdom and philosophy.
~Ludwig van Beethoven

There was no precipitation and, in fact, the sun was shining. At least that is what I was told. I could not see outside. I could see and hear only the faces of strangers who seemed at once both kind and distant as they began to hover around me in increasing numbers. I had just noticed that they all seemed to be wearing white outfits when one of them, the only gentleman in the group, leaned in closer to my face and said, "Good afternoon! How are you feeling today?"

Although I wanted to immediately respond with a heartfelt "I'm fine, thank you, and you?" the words stopped somewhere before my breath could awaken my vocal chords. Suddenly, the idea of saying anything seemed somehow premature since I was gradually realizing that not only did I not know to whom I was speaking, I also did not know where I was. Without an outside view, I could not confirm that it was indeed afternoon or that it was any specific day. I also was at a loss to identify any certain way that I felt as opposed to other ways that I could feel. I certainly could feel no pain but I could not be clear about how I felt about anything else around me.

Through the hushed whispers in the room, I heard unfamiliar electronic sounds. Just as I decided that any attempt at producing an intelligible utterance was not a good plan, I heard a distant female voice say, "He's back with us! He just woke up a moment ago." One by one, the people to my left, who I now recognized as medical staff members, took a half step to one side or the other as the first familiar face appeared.

"Hi, honey!" said my mother as she approached my bedside.

"Why am I here?" I asked as I began to remember that I had classroom assignments due back at the university. I also had to finish preparing for a program that was scheduled to take place at our church, the rehearsal being the reason that I had driven home that Friday.

"Well..." she started out, obviously trying her best to sound calm and reassuring. "Honey, there's been a little accident."

"An accident? Was I in it? Is that why I'm here?" I responded, trying hard to let my voice show more curiosity than anxiety.

"Yes," she said, letting her voice pitch rise just a bit, something she always did when she wanted to let her listener know that there was more to be told.

"Was anyone badly hurt?" I asked, knowing that her answer could either fulfill my worst fears or put them to rest.

Before answering, she looked briefly toward the stethoscope-clad gentleman who had asked the first question. He nodded his approval for her to proceed with more details. Slowly she related the events of the days preceding my awakening, beginning with my departure from the church rehearsal as I headed out onto the highway for the twenty-mile drive back to campus. I was informed that I had been in a coma for two days with a brain injury and a fractured skull resulting from a head-on collision with another car even smaller than my AMC Rambler. It turned out that the other driver had fallen asleep at the wheel, crossed the center line, and suffered injuries nearly identical to my own as he crashed into me on the two-lane highway that connected the two cities.

At first, I was frightened, saddened and depressed that this occurrence might very well leave me with serious and permanent disabilities and could spell the end of my collegiate endeavors—no more singing in choirs and stage shows, no more acting or dancing in stage productions, no more summers teaching swim classes or sitting on lifeguard stands, and I might have to abandon my dreams of becoming a professional performer, completing a music therapy degree, and traveling to other countries.

However, the staff and my dad had other plans. There were two nurses, one of whom could not have been even five feet tall, who daily stood on each side of me while I practiced learning to walk again. After all, my motor skills were a shadow of what they had been before the accident.

No one was more surprised than I when I was able to return to classes after only one week in the hospital. Not only was I able to fully recover and complete my senior year, but my dad accepted an out-of-court settlement that provided enough funds for me to spend the next summer in Europe as a member of the University Division of People-to-People.

I did enter the field of music therapy and eventually became a college professor and published researcher. After extensive study to try to understand my own recovery, I carefully prepared a proposal for a theoretical model designed to explain why brain injury-induced aphasia sufferers recover language skills after participating in music. I was more than surprised when my presentation was accepted for inclusion in a major international conference on music and rehabilitation in New York City. After all, not only was what I was suggesting not mainstream thinking in the world of medicine, it could easily be seen as downright radical since there was absolutely no research to support it. Still, I flew off to the city knowing that if I met too much opposition, I could always play the naïve novice card since the ink on my doctoral diploma had been dry for less than a year.

My short talk included hand-drawn brain diagrams projected onto a screen. To my surprise, my presentation was met with great enthusiasm, as it appeared that the medical professionals in attendance seemed to have been searching for a way to understand the phenomenon of speech recovery following music participation. I had suggested that music helps the brain engage in what I decided to call "functional plasticity," a process that has since been confirmed through research and has replaced the old "abuse it and lose it" brain theory of a quarter century ago. Consequently, I now travel to all corners of the earth speaking about the use of music to stimulate neuroplasticity in brain injury patients.

Although I could not have realized it at the time, the car crash provided direction and a solid foundation for the rest of my academic and professional life. What seemed at first to be a tragic occurrence, I now see as a blessing and I am more than thankful it occurred.

~Dale B. Taylor

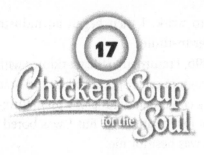

Taking Action

All good writing is like swimming underwater holding your breath.

~F. Scott Fitzgerald

On May 21, 1995, my life changed completely when I was involved in a near-fatal bicycle accident in Scotch Plains, New Jersey. I don't remember much, only riding by a local cemetery; the rest is a blank. I was air lifted to Morristown Memorial Hospital. After undergoing multiple surgeries, I remained in a coma for two days. I awoke to many wires and tubes attached to my body, but also to my family at my bedside.

In addition to my many bodily injuries, I also suffered a traumatic brain injury. Though I thought my life was over, I had actually embarked on a never-ending journey. Weeks later I was discharged and admitted to the Kessler Institute in East Orange, New Jersey. Though I am unable to remember everything about my month-long stay there, I do remember my employer, friends, and family coming to visit me and meeting people who were in the same predicament as I was.

Once I was released from Kessler's inpatient program, my brother asked me to come live with him for a few weeks. During that time I started attending an outpatient program at Kessler consisting of physical and cognitive therapy to help me return to society.

In late November of 1995, I completed my cognitive program and a month later was released from physical therapy. After months of rehabbing at home, I was interviewed by the division of vocational rehab to return to work. I then began an industrial rehabilitation program at Kessler Institute.

In May of 1996, I returned to the workforce with the assistance of Project Pace, a program once sponsored by the Brain Injury Alliance of New Jersey. My coworkers said it was premature for me to return; others said it was just plain crazy. But I was bored at home and my family thought it was best for me.

That week, I attended my first BIANJ support group meeting and my group leader asked me if I was sure I wanted to return because I did not have to work. But my attitude was to finish what I started and not give up.

At about this time, I also began to write. I've had two books published and I re-learned graphic design. Every year I enter some of my work in a disability art expo, to show people my talents. When I became cognitively better, my support group leader empowered me to become a member of the Council for the Head Injured Community (CHIC). For years I have served at the annual BIANJ seminar, at the Kessler Institute where I did my rehab, and also at CAMP TREK (Together in Recreation, Exploration & Knowledge), BIANJ's week-long residential camp for adults with brain injury.

Months later I became a member of the legislative network, assisting BIANJ to get laws passed that benefit not only people who suffer from brain injury but also those who don't. A year later I became a mentor (a program once sponsored by BIANJ). I would speak with my mentees weekly, listen to their problems, and try to make them feel good about themselves. Every year during brain injury awareness month I have gone to New Jersey's capitol to meet with many lawmakers to help them understand the needs of people with brain injury. In 2009 I received the Merriam Goldman positive achievement award for staying positive and making a difference in the brain-injured community.

My road to recovery has been very difficult and it's a journey with no end. There were many things that helped me and still help me with my recovery, activities such as writing, graphic design, speaking to others about TBI and photography. If I had known that I would cause great heartache to my family that day I went biking, I would have stayed home. But if I had, I never would have discovered this world of brave TBI survivors that I did not know existed.

Throughout the years I've learned a lot about being a TBI survivor. Many are worse off than I am but fight to live their lives to the fullest. It's not only about me but others as well. There are many who don't understand traumatic brain injuries. Many people believe they are indestructible but they're not. Unfortunately, it can happen to anyone.

~Joseph Caminiti

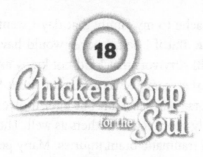

18

Your Voice Sounds Good Today

When words are scarce, they are seldom spent in vain.
~William Shakespeare

Your voice sounds good today." That's what my parents said on the mornings when I was thinking well.

Just over three years ago I hit my head in a car crash. "No big deal," I told the doctor. "I've had eight concussions. I'll be fine."

"No work for three days," he stated. I argued with him that I was on duty as a police officer in two hours. "No work, no driving, and find someone to help with your children for a few days."

My friend came the next day to help with my two foster kids, ages seven and five.

I told her, "The boy did come to the box one time."

Confused, my friend responded that Max was already home.

"No, the boy even now did come one time," I said, trying to explain that Makayla would be home soon.

Improper sentence structure and word choices affected my ability to share my thoughts and feelings with those helping me. I struggled to speak clearly, to understand activities, and experienced strong reactions to sights, sounds, and movements.

The diagnosis was post-concussion syndrome. The brain clinic stated that I had a good chance of a full recovery because I had started therapy so soon after the injury. They suggested that the children leave to give me time to heal.

Three days turned into several months of a hard fight. After ten months of therapy and training, waiting and setbacks, I got my life back. I returned to my road patrol duty. The children returned and I resumed my plan to pursue adoption.

Work was great, at least in short bursts. One morning about a week back into my real life, I answered the phone. "Hi Mom, what even did you want to say to me this morning? I did need to be ready right now to do work."

"Oh, Julie. You need to rest. Your speech and voice aren't good today."

Every aspect of my life was affected. I found that I had to save all of my energy for work. I could only ski a few runs before the movements would cause dizziness. The singing at church was so loud I'd wear earplugs and cover my ears. When my symptoms were obvious to the children, they would tell me to go rest in my room.

If well rested, I did great, my thoughts and responses strong and fast. I could tolerate the pace, sounds, and stress of working and raising children. But the "brain drain" would always return. Sometimes weeks would go by with no symptoms and I would be confident that I was better.

"Your voice doesn't sound good today." Another sick day.

As the year continued, the ups and downs led me to the hardest decision I've ever made.

I held the children close, "I love you two more than life itself. You deserve the best of everything, including a mom who can spend more than a few hours a day with you before resting for work. I love you so much but I can't adopt you."

"But we want you. Don't send us away. We'll be good." They left a few weeks later and were adopted by a wonderful couple.

My heart broke.

Spring came and I still experienced good and bad days. The good stretches became longer and the bad stretches became shorter. My recovery time was more rapid. I began to spend more time with my friends and family. I added activities back into my life outside of work. My fitness improved and two years after my injury I declared myself recovered.

"She hit her head at work tonight," I heard my friend tell my dad. I looked across the hospital room. She spoke into the phone. "No, we don't know how bad it is yet."

I convinced the doctor I was fine and returned to work three days later. I thought I was okay. I didn't lose my ability to speak clearly. I didn't have the visible symptoms I had with the first brain injury. But everything became more difficult. I returned to spending my free time resting, and yet the workdays became longer and harder.

My brain fatigued much more quickly after my on-duty concussion. At the first sign of compromised abilities, I would call in sick.

"My brain feels like a bucket with a hole in it. No matter how much water I put into it, by the end of the day it's empty. I can't get the bucket full enough to last through my shift," I complained to God, begging Him to plug up the hole.

My dad and I went sailing during my 4th of July vacation. It was a wonderful getaway until my dad started a serious conversation. "You need to quit work. It terrifies me that you get disoriented and confused, that you might not be able to react fast enough. It makes me sad that you have to give up everything else so that you can make it through a few shifts at the police department without leaving early."

My vacation became one of heartbreak. I felt that everything I had worked for was gone. I had fought so hard to get back and I had failed. I questioned my own abilities; I thought that if I could just try harder, I'd get better.

My first day back to work from vacation went well. A week of rest was just what I needed. The police calls came in fast and I responded just as quickly. "I don't have to quit," I decided confidently. I started my next shift by taking my cruiser through a car wash. The sounds and movements made me throw up.

"I need to leave." My captain looked at me with sadness in his eyes. "My brain just isn't consistently rested enough to be safe on the job."

A week later I collided with my nephew while playing in the waves. The sand swayed under my feet as my mom helped me stumble to the car.

"Mom, I did even hit my head right now." Back to square one. Hospitals, brain therapy, pacing activities.

I struggled to understand. I was so angry at God for taking away my foster kids, my job, and my capabilities. I was angry that I couldn't do all of the activities I loved. I felt loss after loss. Yet I still trusted Him to use me in a meaningful way and give me a fulfilling life.

I still feel the hurts and losses of the past three years. I still roller coaster with good and bad brain days. But over the past year, I relaxed into life and redefined my priorities. I strengthened my relationships with family and friends. Snowshoeing replaced skiing. I sold my motorcycle and started hiking extensively with my dog. Even though I couldn't sustain being a long-term foster parent myself, I now provide respite for other foster parents. And even though I could not sustain a full-time job as a police officer, I now work as a probation surveillance officer and a private investigator with a flexible schedule.

Today my life is not defined by my head injury. The injury is just a piece of the puzzle and not the complete picture of me.

Life is different now.

And most days I can say, "My voice sounds good today."

~Julie Sanderson

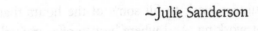

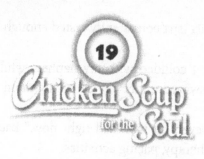

19

Chicken Soup for the Soul

Unexpected Blessings

The unthankful heart... discovers no mercies; but let the thankful heart
sweep through the day and, as the magnet finds the iron, so it will find,
in every hour, some heavenly blessings!
~Henry Ward Beecher

n half an hour I had a diagnosis—post-concussive syndrome—a "mild" traumatic brain injury. When this happens to you, it feels anything but mild. I had fallen headfirst over my bicycle handlebars eighteen months earlier, but since I was wearing a helmet the emergency room doctor never suspected a concussion. Finally, after complaining about cognitive issues for eighteen months, I was at Spaulding Rehabilitation Hospital for diagnosis and care. In conjunction with my brain injury, I had chronic pain and was unable to work; I was on long-term disability and social security.

I had learned the value of hard work, perseverance, and being thankful for the blessings in life from my late mother. I took these values and pursued volunteer work to fill some of the hours that were left empty from not working. And where best to offer my volunteer time and commitment than the Brain Injury Association of Massachusetts (BIA-MA)? I felt that they would understand my cognitive issues and would offer me volunteer projects that would value my strengths versus my weaknesses, weaknesses I felt every day from my brain injury. This volunteer work provided me the opportunity to leave my house and socialize, stay up-to-date on computer applications, feel self-confident again, and succeed, even if the victories were small.

In 2011 I had another fall, tripping over a garden hose and falling face first onto the driveway. This fall exacerbated my pain, and my cognitive issues continued. But with three years of volunteering under my belt, I felt confident in my ability to work again, and began my quest to return to work full-time. The staff at BIA-MA made me feel valued and appreciated for any and all help that I gave to them, no matter the project. The manager of volunteers, Patty Carlson, was tremendous in offering me support and mentoring.

Volunteering helped me learn that I could still perform tasks I had done prior to my brain injury and that despite my pain, work was possible. Work was actually a great distraction from my pain and from one big side effect of my brain injury, "brain chatter," when I hear my voice talking and singing and I have weird thoughts as if I am dreaming.

In October of 2012 I was offered a paid position at the BIA-MA. I continue to successfully work there today because I value the importance of having a job and working hard every day. I enjoy the relationships with my supportive colleagues, and my self-esteem and confidence grow every day I go to the office. I have no doubt that these experiences are helping my brain to heal.

I have been able to end my reliance on social security through the Ticket to Work program and no longer receive checks. I am thrilled and proud every time I get my paycheck from BIA-MA.

Traumatic brain injury, for me, became a valuable learning experience and an unexpected gift. I never look back at my accidents in anger and I see the many blessings I have received because of them, as many wonderful people, places, and experiences have graced my life since that first fall.

~Sandra A. Madden

Chapter
3

Recovering *from* Traumatic Brain Injuries

Never Giving Up

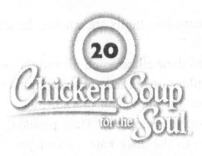

20

After the Dark Clouds, Contentment

Clouds come floating into my life, no longer to carry rain or usher storm,
but to add color to my sunset sky.
~Rabindranath Tagore

I looked at my husband in his hospital bed. His swollen head was bound in bandages and his eyes were closed, but he was no longer in a coma. A retired university law professor, he had gone from lecturing large classes to not speaking at all.

Full of questions, and needing reassurance, I asked the doctor, "When will he be able to walk and talk again?" He looked at me and answered, "Ask me that a year from now." I thought his answer was cold, but I know now that he was just being honest. He gave me no false hope, but instead a bit of advice: "When you pray, don't ask God for anything. Just thank Him for today." That wasn't the way I usually prayed. I brought God all my worries, wants and needs, but the doctor's advice made sense. God already knew what I needed.

Our problems began one August night when my husband fell in the kitchen and hit his head. Weeks later he walked slower and staggered. One evening in September, he leaned down to put books on a low shelf and crumpled to the floor. We rushed him to the hospital. An MRI showed a blood clot pressing on his brain. Surgery was performed and the clot removed, but the bleeding didn't stop. After a second surgery, the surgeon came out with a solemn face.

"The next twenty-four hours are crucial," he said. "I'm not going back in there again."

I knew he had done all he could do and the rest was up to God.

Our grandchildren recorded encouraging messages. We placed the tape player on his pillow and played it every day hoping their voices would help him wake up. They pleaded, "Please wake up, Pepa. We can't go to the State Fair without you." "Pepa, I wonder what you're thinking right now." "I love you, Pepa."

Deep in my inner being I knew my husband would survive. I couldn't imagine life without him. The first glimmer of hope came when my husband was in the process of getting a feeding tube inserted into his stomach. In the recovery room, I held his hand. He squeezed my finger. It was his first physical response, and I felt that a miracle had just happened. Soon afterward he was transferred to an acute-care hospital. There, two therapists lifted him to a sitting position on the side of his bed. When I saw his head fall limply to his chest, my heart sank. Devastated, I thought, "He can't even lift his head. Is this how it's going to be?" I left the room sobbing.

In time, he made more progress physically, then mentally, and our family was elated when he was accepted at a rehab hospital in Dallas for brain-injured patients. There he worked on his speech, memory and comprehension. When he became frustrated with his inability to talk, he gritted his teeth and growled. But his therapy would soon be postponed.

In December, an MRI showed a new bleed, which meant another surgery. I hoped this would be the last, wondering how much more he could stand. When he was finally out of intensive care and in a private room, I was allowed to stay with him. Now, maybe he would get better and resume therapy. Dark clouds hovered over Dallas, and a major ice storm enveloped the city for days. Going home and back would have been impossible. I prayed and wrote poetry.

Then, my husband suffered a stroke. I couldn't believe it. The entire time I had been hoping and praying that he would be able to continue his therapy. When he was re-evaluated for therapy, he failed the test. He couldn't understand a simple command: "Point to the floor." If he was at his lowest moment, so was I. Weeping and praying, I wondered what would happen next. At this point he was dependent on a feeding tube for food in and a catheter for urine out.

When we admitted him into a skilled-nursing facility near our home, I felt we were giving up. Every day I cried on my way there and cried when I left. I had a towel in my car to catch my tears. I tried to deny it, but I was depressed. When friends asked how he was doing, I dropped my head and tears stung my eyes. It was hard for me to talk about it. After fifty-five years of marriage, our roles had completely reversed. He, who was strong and in charge, became weak; I, the weaker one and a follower, became strong and more independent.

Finally, there was a major breakthrough when he remembered his family. One day he asked, "Why did you leave me?" I assured him that I had been there every day. Gradually, the dark clouds of that bitter cold winter passed, and our future seemed hopeful.

There were gaps in his memory, and his speech was far from perfect, but he began to make progress. He didn't remember that he ever had a feeding tube or a catheter, but he recalled his childhood. What he had forgotten, we replaced by making new memories.

During my visits now, we often sit in the courtyard under the gazebo. We watch cardinals build their nest in a Rose of Sharon bush. Silver airplanes glide through the sky on their way to Love Field or DFW Airport. My husband notices the vapor contrails left by high-flying jets, and watches them spread and fade away.

He, who was an avid reader, can no longer hold a book. The entire right side of his body was affected by the surgeries and stroke. He enjoys hearing me read though, and within one year we read through the entire Bible together. Sometimes he attends the scheduled activities, but television and radio are favorites. He handles his wheelchair well and wheels himself around faster than I can walk. A highlight in his routine is when our daughter takes him out to eat, and sometimes to a movie. He looks forward to those outings.

When I remember him over six years ago in a coma, and I see his amazing progress, I feel we are blessed. As the Apostle Paul said in Philippians, "I have learned the secret of being content in any and every situation," my husband and I are learning contentment with our situation. I know that God is in control, and when I pray, I always remember the words of the doctor as I say, "Thank you God for today."

~Betty B. Cantwell

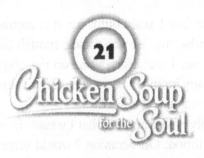

21

It's Worth Fighting For

Permanence, perseverance and persistence in spite of all obstacles,
discouragements and impossibilities: It is this that in all things
distinguishes the strong soul from the weak.

~Thomas Carlyle

I was your average six-year-old boy without problems or worries. The world was mine and I lived with a hunger for knowledge. On my walks home from school I took the scenic way, despite my mother's protests that I had to cross two streets. In the town of Kirkland Lake, Ontario, with 9,000 people, you were lucky to even see a car drive by. I enjoyed my walks and discovered the world for myself a little bit at a time.

I have no memory of that day or even that week. All I recall is seeing the ceiling of an ambulance and a flurry of activity around me. I had been struck by a truck going thirty miles per hour. How fortunate I was to be alive. My local hospital was not equipped to handle my broken body and sent me off to Sault St. Marie, Ontario. Despite the severity of the accident, I only sustained a broken femur, collarbone and mild fractures of my neck, all of which simply needed time to heal. However I did get headaches often and falling asleep was strangely difficult. After a two-month stay in the hospital, I had finally healed enough and was ready to get home and play with friends.

School wasn't like I remembered. Everything seemed so difficult. It was as if I had forgotten everything. My body cast was replaced with a wheelchair but I still could not run around with everyone. After several months, my leg was strong enough to play but no one would play with me. I was often alone on the playground. The constant teasing and my inability to understand the simplest concepts in school made me sad and confused.

It hurts deeply now, knowing that I wasn't the only one suffering through my childhood. On occasion I would remark to my parents that I wanted to die—drown myself in the public pool and be done with it. My strongest wish, I told my mother, was to turn into a toy; that way I could exist without the knowledge of living or the pain of emotions. It was my way of saying something was wrong with me though I didn't know what. I can't imagine the heartache and helplessness they must have felt at my remarks and calls for help.

I transferred schools. The new students were worse. They took a strange happiness in their ability to exclude me and steal my things while the teacher screamed. After another year I was forced to do strange tests with grown-ups. The tests went something like this: What do you see? What's wrong with this picture? I enjoyed them because I was taken out of the class and asked questions I could actually answer. My mother sat me down one day and told me that I had suffered a traumatic brain injury from the accident. My brain was bruised and there really wasn't a cure. That meant very little to me then; after all I had just failed third grade.

Ms. Brand, my first special needs teacher, taught me how to read and write again. For the first time, I met someone who understood my condition and was able to give me hope. After an entire summer, seven days a week, for three hours a day, I could learn and understand school again. However it wasn't enough.

The next few years were a blur. My family moved away from Kirkland in pursuit of special needs programs for me. I had many teachers and therapists with little success. In my eleventh year I met an interesting lady named Mrs. Price, a highly educated special needs tutor. She gave me the ability to truly learn again. For years on end she forced knowledge into my brain until it ached. She gave me the platform to grab onto and rebuild myself. For the first time in my life I had a direction, the willpower, and ability to learn and move forward on my own.

I still have migraines and sleep problems. My brain injury is on the frontal lobe, the part that makes you, you. I was no longer the same person after my accident. I understand now that my classmates were too young to understand what had happened to me and why I was different. It even took the professionals two years to diagnose my condition. Having a better understanding of my condition might have helped. I now know why I suffered like I did for the first five years after my accident and am able to forgive those who don't even remember me anymore.

Today I am twenty-five and in my last year of college. Every day I am thankful for what I have and where I am. Every day I continue to recover from my TBI. I will myself to stay strong and confident and I find happiness with my family and the friends I have managed to make at college.

Persistence. That is the only advice I can give. There is no easy way. Push yourself. Force your way through despite everything and harden your mind against the negative. You are you and that is something extraordinary. Grind your mind, body and soul to their limits and overcome whatever stands in your way.

I wanted to give up: ignore school and just stay in a bottomless hole. My parents dragged me around, refusing to give up on me when I gave up on myself. They had the power and willingness to push me when I would not push myself. I would not be where I am now without them. To those not blessed with people to push you, push yourself. Carve your own way through life, fighting with everything you have. After all, it's your life you're fighting for.

~Tyler Tatasciore

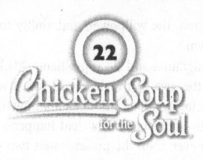

Waiting for John to Remember

Music in the soul can be heard by the universe.

~Lao Tzu

My son John loved to play hockey. It was a big part of his life, even when he was little. And it didn't matter where the game was—in the driveway with boys from the neighborhood, knee hockey in the kitchen, in the basement.

John played ice hockey for the local travel team. He enjoyed the excitement and challenge of the game and being in the locker room with his friends. While I worried about John playing hockey, I was reassured that the peewee division banned checking.

On December 1, 2012, when he was eleven years old, John sustained a traumatic brain injury. In a short-handed play, John cleared the puck from his defensive zone. His teammate picked it up near center ice and rushed for a breakaway. An opposing player didn't like that, and went after John. I watched in disbelief as the opponent came up behind John and used his elbow deliberately and strongly to hit my son's head into the boards.

"Johnny!" My heart raced as I banged on the glass of the ice rink. John fell backward and hit his head again on the ice. This couldn't be happening. And it never should have happened in a non-checking division, especially when John didn't have possession of the puck.

I knew this was bad. I had watched my sons play hockey for ten years, and seen them fall on the ice. But this time was different. The coaches helped him off the ice and sat him on the bench. I immediately ran to his side. I wanted him out of the game.

I wanted to believe that John wasn't hurt as badly as it appeared. He seemed dazed, but he was conscious. He told me his head hurt a lot and I was scared. His eyes were widely dilated and I knew that was a bad sign. But the emergency pediatrician in the evening clinic didn't seem alarmed. She said he had a concussion and to watch him. So we did.

The next day we had tickets for a show in the city and we went. But John started acting strangely. He couldn't walk well and he leaned against the walls of the theater for support. I called his regular pediatrician when we got home and made an appointment for the next day.

John's symptoms worsened. By the time he arrived in the doctor's office, he had no interest in anything. He was confused and withdrawn. The doctor performed basic neurological tests. I knew we had a serious issue when John couldn't recite the months of the year backward from December. He couldn't remember what came before October. There were other clues, too. I offered to make scrambled eggs for him one morning a few days after his injury.

"Please get some eggs from the refrigerator for me," I asked.

"Sure," John said. But he paused by the door and asked, "What does an egg look like?"

I tried not to look shocked, but I was starting to panic.

I thought all he had to do was rest and he would be back to normal in a week or two. Unfortunately, I wasn't yet aware how "not normal" our lives would become during the following month. I watched helplessly as we discovered how seriously impacted John's brain was. Within the next two weeks, his condition continued to deteriorate instead of improve. John couldn't recognize familiar people or places. He couldn't recall basic factual information. It was alarming that he didn't know that the inside of an oven was hot, an electric outlet was dangerous, or what the difference was between "real" food and toy, or "fake," food. He didn't remember much of anything prior to his injury.

It frightened us to see the extent of his amnesia. In his actions and abilities, John seemed to have regressed to the level of a five-year-old boy.

I continued to talk to his pediatrician on a daily basis, but quickly looked for a pediatric neurologist. Finding someone who had seen a case like John's was difficult. A few doctors suggested that he was malingering and that these symptoms couldn't be happening from a concussion. John had an MRI and it showed normal brain structure, which was somewhat reassuring. But the memory loss persisted and he was clearly unable to function at a sixth-grade level. John couldn't go to school. At this point he was reading kindergarten level books, although he preferred that I read them to him. He lost even the most basic math skills. Friends came to visit. He had no idea who some of them were. John was also easily startled and refused to walk along the sidewalks, fearing that the passing cars on the street would hit him.

I spent most of the first three weeks crying, devastated. I was angry, angry that this happened to John and to us. I wanted to find the kid who hit him and let him know what he did to all of us. But most of all, I desperately wanted my son back. This was no longer the person we knew and loved. John spent most of that time staring vacantly—and humming music—and that was the only thing that linked us to his past.

We have a musical household. John and his brothers play violin and all listen to the classical music station on the radio daily. John absentmindedly hummed tunes he played years ago. Bits of melody swirled around inside his head and seemed to comfort him as he played with his Legos, the only other thing he could still do. It was Christmastime and the radio played Christmas carols and songs. John memorized the words to every single one he heard.

Then he started to play the piano, which might not sound strange except that he hadn't played since kindergarten. John picked out his Vivaldi violin concerto on the piano perfectly. It was bizarre, but it made him happy and seeing him happy made us happy too. After four weeks, I gave him the violin again. Although he could not identify the numbered measures on the orchestral score, he could still read music and play the violin. Just before the injury, he was accepted into Westchester's All-County Orchestra with a concert in three months. I am happy to say that he participated in the performance. Having the music definitely helped his recovery.

Unlike a broken bone, there isn't much to do for a brain injury but wait and pray. Two months after his injury, he returned to school on a part-time basis. Mostly, he sat in classes and observed. His teachers realized he couldn't do homework and stopped sending it home. They reported seeing him as a significantly different person in the classroom compared with prior to the injury. We all waited for John to heal. John's friends were loyal and helped him every day in school to relearn normal activities (such as finding his classroom and opening his locker.) The school district also made accommodations for him. Three months after his injury, he was able to tell me stories about his day in school. But he still couldn't do the homework. It was practically June before John made progress in school. He had tutors after school and throughout the summer to help him relearn or remember things he needed to know.

It is now eleven months since John's injury. He looks like an ordinary seventh- grade student, walking to school and doing his homework and enjoying the company of his friends. There are still pieces missing from his past, and occasionally he asks questions that remind me that there are things he still cannot recall. But for the most part, life is good for him and that makes us all very grateful.

I always had faith that we would find a way for John to reconnect his life again. I never gave up hope that he would recover and thrive once more. I wished I could have met someone who had experienced amnesia so we would have known what to expect. In writing this, I hope I can inspire someone else to believe that they or their loved one will improve too.

~Anita Dziwura

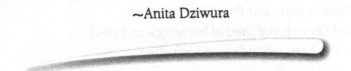

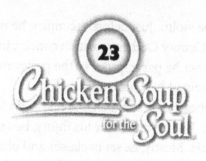

23

Anguish

Courage is not simply one of the virtues,
but the form of every virtue at the testing point.
~C.S. Lewis

An eternity of anguish changes nothing
Nothing prepares you for unconscious
Unconscious saved by the Jaws of Life
The Jaws of Life get you to the emergency room
The emergency room continues saving your life
When your life is ready for ICU
You're told what happened
And that your name is Richard
From your lack of response
They understand that you understand
Nothing

Eighteen tons of cement truck didn't stop at the stop
Fracturing my hand and my hip
Damaging my equilibrium
My jaw, my teeth, my vision, my brain, my spine

Thirteen years and I'm still in recovery
And I'm sick and tired of being sick and tired
So I've been rebuilding and refueling

Refueling and retooling
Self-teaching self-schooling
Relearning how to walk, talk and think

Mood shifts and concentration declines
Hands shake and head pounds
Or you become anxious and confused
My hip dips and my foot slips
My jaw clicks and my brain sticks

All because one day
You leave the house to run three miles
Then go to the gym to work out
The next day you leave the house for work
And go by ambulance to the emergency room
Kissing your fifteen-year telecom career and your health
Goodbye

On any given day breathing is not an option

Surviving the accident was easy
Living the rest of my life
Became my greatest challenge

So I leave you with this message
Whatever trouble you may have
Or whatever it is that makes you, you
Or the person you want to be
Don't ever, under any circumstance
Consider the possibility of giving up
If I gave up I wouldn't be here

Adversity knows no boundaries
And neither should we

Because an eternity of anguish
Changes nothing

~Richard E. Berg

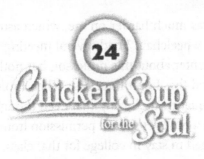

24

Graduating from College

A dream doesn't become a reality through magic; it takes sweat, determination, and hard work.

~Colin Powell

As my sister helped slip my graduation gown over my head, I remembered when I first attended Sussex County Community College back in 1998, five years after my traumatic brain injury that started with a fall I took two days before ACL surgery. Even after five years of speech therapy three times a week, my speech was still not 100% understandable, so when I decided to sign up for English 101, I couldn't help thinking, "Is this a big mistake?"

When my aide first pushed my wheelchair into the classroom, I wasn't sure if I would be able to speak or not. Would I get the words in my sentences all mixed up like I usually did? I also worried that I did not have a college-level vocabulary, so I was afraid I wouldn't be able to understand the work. I had e-mailed my professor, Gary Mielo, prior to class to explain my traumatic brain injury and my deficits, including my speech difficulties. I shared with him my doubts about my ability to succeed in college. He wrote back, saying it would be an honor to have me as a student who is fighting back from a brain injury. My love for learning and my determination helped get me through that class with a 4.0.

My professor encouraged me to take another class the following semester, so I signed up for English 102 with a different professor.

This professor was much harder on me, which astonished me, since she too was in a wheelchair. I had several meetings with the director of the learning center about this professor, but nothing was resolved. I was so frustrated that I quit the class. When Professor Mielo heard about this, he e-mailed me saying that even though he wasn't teaching that class, he would get special permission from the Dean to tutor me online. I agreed to stay in college for that class, as long as he was my professor.

With my hunger for knowledge, I thought I was soaking up facts like a sponge, but I was frustrated that by the following day I would often have no memory of what I'd learned. I spent most of my time with a tutor in the learning center; I figured if I was going to be in college and spend my time and money on that class, then I wanted an A in it. When the semester ended, I had earned that A, and again Professor Mielo talked me into taking another class, and another, then another until he finally convinced me to go for my degree. Professor Mielo became my advisor and mentor until he retired in 2011.

Fifteen years later, here I was, standing in the front of the line, ready to lead all the students into the tent for graduation. This was not in the rehearsal, so what a surprise it was for me! Dressed in my cap and gown with the honor tassel dangling from my cap and Phi Theta Kappa gold and blue cords, I realized how many people I had proven wrong.

I thought back to nineteen years before, when I woke up in the intensive care unit on a ventilator with tubing and wires attached to my body. I couldn't move my right side or talk. I didn't remember anything.

Back then, when people talked to me, it sounded like a cassette tape on fast-forward, all jumbled up. I spent over thirty days in a private room at the hospital with the same doctor coming in, asking me the same questions over and over, "Who is the President? What day is it? What year is it?"

One morning, I remembered the nurses were saying that Hillary was President. I did not know who Hillary was, but I scribbled down her name on my table. The doctor came in and asked me who the

President was and I replied, "Hillary." He said, "No, Hillary is not the President." But I insisted, "Hillary." Again, I said, "Hillary," thinking maybe I didn't pronounce her name correctly and he said, "No." I was getting upset and finally started pointing towards the nurse's station, yelling, "Them say, them say!" He went to the nurse's station to find out why I was getting upset and pointing towards the nurses. The nurses told him that they had been kidding around earlier, saying how Hillary ran the country, not mentioning that Bill Clinton was the President. The doctor informed the nurses that if they were going to joke around, to close my door, because I was insisting that Hillary was the President of the United States.

The sound of bagpipes snapped me back to the present and I started to march slowly into the huge tent, leading the other graduates behind me. I made my way to my reserved seat at the end of the second row. I never thought I would see this day happen when I started back in 1998. Although my back was throbbing in pain and at times I thought I would be sick to my stomach from the Vicodin, I forced myself to push forward, putting one foot in front of the other without my cane or braces. This was one of the proudest moments in my life.

I am so very thankful to the many people who have been by my side, my family and friends especially. I am particularly grateful to Gary Mielo, my first college professor, the staff and therapists at Progressive Health of New Jersey, and my therapy team at Rehabilitation Specialists, where I continue my treatment today. I am indebted to everyone who gave me the confidence to continue making strides, large and small. Their support, along with my own determination, have brought me to this point.

~Donna Fitzpatrick

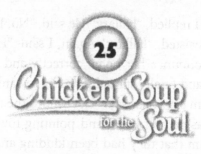

25

Healing Your Heart
after a Brain Injury

We are human "beings", not human "doings."
~Bernie Siegel, MD

When a car skidded into mine on a slippery road in 1991, I felt very lucky. Although my car was totaled, I had my seatbelt on and I didn't have a scratch on me. I had blacked out only for a moment and I looked okay. The emergency room sent me home with instructions to take Advil.

I thought that I couldn't think because I was exhausted and in so much pain. I had a severe case of whiplash. I could barely eat or talk. As I slowly healed physically, I began to realize that I couldn't do anything mentally that I used to do effortlessly. I was a wife and mother and I managed the household. I had worked professionally in teaching, banking and healthcare. I was an achiever; multitasking, problem solving and organizing were second nature to me. Now I couldn't remember what I was doing. I couldn't figure out what to wear. I couldn't find my words. I couldn't follow the storyline while reading to my son or watching TV. I was a bank officer and I literally could not hold 2 + 2 in my head long enough to get 4. I had lived in town for twenty years and I couldn't find my way around. I had been a home economics/consumer science teacher and I couldn't cook supper. Noise and confusion overwhelmed me.

My brain used to feel like a fancy multi-function machine,

copying, sorting and collating all at once. Now, the harder I tried to do what I used to do, the more meltdowns and shutdowns I had. I thought I was losing my mind. I remember thinking "this must be what going crazy feels like." I wasn't feeling so lucky anymore.

Eventually, I found help. It took time, it was the hardest work I have ever done, and it changed my life forever.

Something essential that I learned and wish I'd known during this journey is that there is usually a grieving process associated with healing from a brain injury. I learned that there are common stages associated with the grieving process: denial, anger, bargaining, depression, and acceptance. I also learned that processing grief is not a straightforward path. One typically moves back and forth in the different stages and that is normal. I learned that in order to heal and be able to move forward, it is necessary to recognize your feelings, acknowledge the losses, allow yourself to feel the feelings and mourn the losses.

The devastating losses brain injury survivors experience are far-reaching. On top of struggling with physical injuries and cognitive deficits, there are usually secondary losses as well: income, jobs, social networks, friends, even family and homes. Survivors often lose parts of their lives that took years, sometimes even decades, to build. Something else to consider is that your family and friends may be grieving too. When you think about it, they have lost the person you used to be and the role you used to play in their lives as well.

Needless to say, the changes and losses I experienced had a profound effect on me, on my being. I found myself struggling with a fundamental life crisis: who am I and what is my value if I can't do what I used to do, if my friends aren't my friends anymore and I'm a problem for my family? I had lost my self-confidence and my sense of self. I was becoming more and more depressed. I contemplated suicide.

Getting in touch with my spiritual guides was instrumental in helping me move through the grieving process and heal my heart. I needed to hear that I had value in my being, not just in my doing. Being part of a support group for brain injury survivors let me know I was not alone in my struggle.

One of the keys for me was to forgive myself for not being able to do what I used to be able to do. I also needed to forgive others for their shortcomings. Ignoring your feelings will hold you back. Your grief and whatever way it manifests in your life will create stress and inhibit your rehabilitation process overall. Our brains work best when we feel well, physically and emotionally.

Here are some suggestions to help you heal your heart:

- Keep a gratitude journal, writing down three things every day that were successful, an improvement, or made you smile.
- Arrange regular get-togethers with friends, even if just to chat on the phone or to meet for a cup of coffee or tea.
- Spend some time on a hobby.
- Practice random acts of kindness.
- Volunteer.
- Get some physical exercise, every day.
- Go outdoors; soak up some fresh air, sunshine and vitamin D.
- Sign up for a class, anything that interests you.
- Think about what is most important to you and how you can bring more of it into your life.
- Keep your perspective, refer to your calendar and journals to look back and note improvements. Celebrate what you can do now that you couldn't do six months or a year ago.
- Remember that you are still the same unique and valuable person inside, with the same loves that you had before your injury. No injury can take that away from you.

Today, my brain can work like that fancy copy machine again when conditions are optimal. I can do quality work again if I plan it, allowing extra time for fatigue and "bad brain days." I have rebuilt skills and regained stamina. I am able to listen to my intuition. I can depend on myself again. Hallelujah!

Today I am a lucky lady! I have had the privilege of facilitating an amazing Brain Injury Survivor Support Group since 1995. I work for the Brain Injury Association of Massachusetts, assisting other support groups. I have also written a book, a collection of "brain injury survivor wisdom," to help other survivors. My mission is to encourage survivors to continue their healing process, to never give up, to inspire hope. Healing from a brain injury shouldn't stop just because your insurance coverage does. You never know what the future may hold and how much you can recover.

~Barbara J. Webster

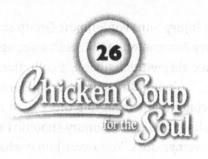
Yes, I'm a Train Wreck

Gird your hearts with silent fortitude, suffering yet hoping all things.
~Felicia Hemans

Most people in upstate New York remember March 15, 1993 as the day the blizzard of the century paralyzed our region. That day had a profound impact on me, too, but not for the reasons you may think.

The place where I worked after school had closed down early that day. The storm was coming fast, dumping six inches of wet snow in less than an hour. It was five o'clock and I was glad to be heading home early. At eighteen years old, I didn't care too much about the impending storm. March meant spring was finally here, and the only thing I was thinking about was graduating from high school in a few short months. My grades had put me at the top of my class and I had just been accepted into engineering college, a hard-earned dream come true. I was on the swim team, played in the orchestra, and had a girlfriend. From my perspective, eighteen was the best age ever. I didn't have a worry in the world.

As I headed out of work that day, I glanced up toward the gray sky that hung low over the town. I couldn't see much in front of me, just the thick snowflakes that stung my face and mounded quickly around my feet. The wind was relentless so I flipped my coat collar up high, put on my headphones, and headed down the road. In hindsight, I guess this is the place where I went wrong. But it all seemed innocent enough at the time. I turned the music up full blast and strongly considered taking the forbidden shortcut home along the back railroad tracks. It would be okay, I reasoned. After all, the news report said a state of emergency had been declared, meaning the trains couldn't possibly be running, right? I decided to go for it. I sneaked up over the back bank and walked out onto the blustery trail, the metal train tracks guiding my way home already invisible. It was getting worse outside, but no big deal. My house was only a few minutes away.

The music blaring from my headphones was so loud that I didn't hear the warning blast of the train whistle. The snow was blinding me and muffling the sounds around me. It wasn't until my feet rattled beneath me that I turned around. Looming over my head was the face of a huge, black metal train, staring down at me through the dusk. With no time to think, I did the only thing I could do. I jumped high in the air and tried to get out of the way.

That's it. That's the last thing I remember of the blizzard of the century. One mistaken decision, one rumble from the ground, one flash of black in the storm, and my life was changed forever.

I learned about the rest of my ordeal from my parents. They learned about it from the people who witnessed the accident and its aftermath. The conductor said I bounced three times off the front of the train before I was tossed into the air like a rag doll. The police officer said I was thrown fifty feet from the railroad track. The emergency response team said they searched much of the night before finally finding me, unconscious, buried in three feet of snow. The doctor told my parents that I would be dead before morning.

My dad was a minister who believed strongly in the power of prayer. I'm not sure why God decided I should stay here on this planet. Maybe it was because of the people from all of the different countries who prayed for me that night. I don't know. All I know for sure is that my dad started a prayer chain that began at my hospital bed and traveled around the world and reached as far away as China. I made it through that night, and the next night, and the night after that. The doctor just shook his head, telling my parents not to get their hopes up. I still might not make it and if I did I might remain in a permanent vegetative state. But live I did. And seven months later, I emerged from my deep coma wondering what the heck hit me.

"A train." my mother said. "You were hit by a train."

"Who gets hit by a train?" I asked her. I truly thought my family and friends were playing some kind of joke on me. Unfortunately, the doctor echoed her words and that's when the denial set in. It couldn't be as bad as they were saying. Never walk again? Never swim or use my arms or hands? Memory and speech problems? They were all liars. My life would go back to normal and it would happen soon. But soon didn't happen. After months in rehab, I reluctantly realized they were telling me the truth. For the next thirteen months, I would fight to keep depression and anger from suffocating me.

I went through a long stretch of time when I was mad at everyone: my parents, the doctors, even God. What gave them the right to decide for me that I should stay on this planet and work so hard—just to regain a small semblance of my old life? I wasn't so sure that I wanted to stay! And I wasn't so sure I wanted to be the guy whose identity was stolen by a beaten up brain and body. I had to learn how to talk, how to eat, and even how to breathe—a shock to a kid who was on the swim team. My lungs had multiple punctures in them, to the point where I swear I could hear the "wind" whistle when I took a deep breath. I couldn't even sit up without support. I called myself the blob because it took months for me to regain the use of my torso muscles. Nothing worked right anymore. But worst of all, my life didn't work anymore either. Facing that fact was the hardest part.

But deep down I am an eternal optimist. Through it all, I hung onto a good-sized chunk of denial, in spite of the reality of my situation. I am grateful for this piece of denial, because without it, I would have fallen into a severe depression, one that I might not have had the wherewithal to climb out of. Actually I may still be living in denial. But that's okay. Brain injury or no brain injury, I am very bright and my deficits aren't going to ruin me. Yeah, so I have a few problems. Who doesn't, right? Now, eighteen years and an entire lifetime later, I still spend my days in a wheelchair. I have poor vision, spasticity in my left arm, and little use of my hands. Just going to the bathroom can be a major ordeal. The doctors still tell me that I will never get better. That is depressing, yes, but I view it this way: never say never! I've made a lot of progress through the years and I intend to keep it up for many years to come.

You might ask what my driving force is, what keeps me going every day in spite of the fact that I am so impaired. It's simple. I stay strong for all of the people who have been strong for me. On rare occasions, when I catch myself wishing that the train did end my life, I think of my friends and family and how it would be for them if I gave up. If I start feeling sorry for myself, I try to remember that a lot of people look up to me. I'm a survivor, not because I want to be, but because I have to be for the benefit of those who see me as an inspiration. I am a reluctant role model.

Many people ask me how to deal with hard issues in their lives, be they physical, emotional, or spiritual. I know they look at me and think, if a train couldn't put him down, nothing can. Then, I think—hell, yeah! I'm a survivor who has used my inner strength to reinvent my life. I go to work every day and have my own apartment. I have many friends and I love to go to restaurants and flirt with the waitresses. And, best of all, I have a sense of humor that makes all those long-faced non-survivors realize that life can be a joy—if you let it. I have a lot of insight to share. If my opinion was pay-worthy, I'd be rich.

This experience has made me realize that I can create my own miracles. I'm still working on staying happy for myself, on being my own motivation. But in spite of it all, I *am* a happy guy. And, I am rich. Wouldn't you agree? I am rich in friends, stamina, and in life.

My life rocks.

~Jon Nathan Blair

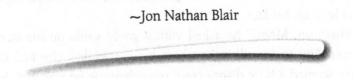

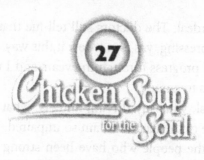

27

Family, Faith, Friends... Can

To gather with God's people in united adoration of the Father is as necessary to the Christian life as prayer.
~Martin Luther

It had, so far, been the worst year of our sixteen-year marriage. We had both recently lost our jobs and a pregnancy we had waited years for. My mother was exhibiting symptoms of ischemic disease and we watched her fail daily. Things just couldn't get much worse, in my estimation.

Then one afternoon, after finishing his paper route, my fourteen-year-old son Chris and his friend began "trick-riding" in front of our home on bicycles that were much too small for them.

Suddenly Chris's friend ran screaming into our home. "Chris fell off his bike, Mrs. Matero! I can't wake him up!" Wayne's voice was hysterical as he told me how Chris had hit a manhole cover and was thrown headfirst onto its cleats.

In a panic I ran into the street just in time to see Chris sitting up, a dazed look on his face.

"What's up, Mom?" he asked with a goofy smile on his face. I convinced him to sit still right where he was while I checked him over. He seemed a little disoriented, but otherwise he was fine. So I thought...

My husband insisted I call our doctor to report that Chris had been knocked unconscious by his fall. I none-too-gently reminded him that we had no insurance; and that Chris was just "bumped up" and not severely injured. Nevertheless, I ended up calling our doctor.

Our family physician insisted we bring him directly to the emergency room, citing the death of a basketball player from a closed head injury just the week before my son's accident. I recalled reading the newspaper account regarding this young man; stating that no one had sought medical attention for him when he fell on the basketball court.

By the time we reached the ER, Chris had become so violent that it took four orderlies to remove him from our car and put him on a transport gurney. He kicked the ER nurse in the jaw so hard she had to seek medical attention herself.

Our doctor met us shortly after Chris had been taken for imaging studies.

"This is bad, guys," he said. "He has a torn blood vessel at the base of his brain. We need to take him to surgery immediately. We have to find it and try to repair it or he may not recover."

As we waited in the waiting room, we suddenly realized that someone had called our church and it wasn't long before we were surrounded by friends holding us up and praying for Chris. In that small, crowded room my husband fell to his knees. Holding up his hands, he prayed. "Lord God, my Father. Please heal my son. Please let him stay with us, Father. I know you gave your only Son, but I can't give mine. You are God, but I'm just a man; and he's my only son. I beg You, don't take my son!" His voice was so plaintive and his prayer so heart-wrenching.

At this time, my brother, an Army officer at Fort Lewis, Washington entered the room. I was shocked to see him here, and so soon. My dad had called him to ask for prayer and he had caught a military flight within minutes of hearing the news. He felt strongly that we needed family support at this time.

The neurosurgeon reported to us that Chris's surgery had gone better than expected, but that his prognosis was uncertain. I begged to be allowed to see my son but I had to wait until the following day.

The next morning when I saw Chris his head was three times its normal size. No one had told me that the head could swell following an invasive surgery and I was scared to death.

"What's up, Mom?" he said. His smile was the old familiar one; and I praised God that my son was still "in there," that he could speak and recognize people. The doctors told us that he might exhibit strange emotional behaviors for some time, and that his coordination might be impaired, but we didn't care. God had spared our son!

We were so happy that Chris had survived that we didn't give much thought to how we would pay all the expense, even though we had no jobs and no insurance. We realized after seeing what God had done for Chris that He would do the same for us if we only trusted Him.

During his recovery at home, Chris's boss at the newspaper came to see us. He told us Chris had an insurance policy that would cover the amount our major insurance carrier didn't pay. When I told him that we had no insurance, he said they would cover everything. It seems that Chris had signed up for full insurance coverage accidently, and had never gotten around to adjusting it to the more pared-down version, as he had intended to.

Our family, friends, and our entire faith community spent the next few weeks ministering to us in any way they could. We received gifts of meals, food for our pantry and our freezer, money for additional expenses, and moral support beyond measure. My brother, who owned the house we lived in, would not take rent money from us until Chris had fully recovered. We counted the number of states and foreign countries where prayers were being offered for him via prayer chains requested by our family and friends. It was truly humbling to know that the globe was literally encircled with prayer for him.

Chris suffered no physical problems from his accident. In addition to the torn blood vessel, there was damage to his prefrontal cortex from the impact of his fall. He has experienced some behavioral difficulties from that. He has rare, but definite problems with impulse control; and when greatly agitated, his reasoning skills revert emotionally to the age he was when injured.

It was not always easy for us or for those around him. We learned that his behavior was usually injury-connected and not willful. That made it easier for us to overlook some of his outbursts and help him through it, rather than correcting him. As he has matured, his problems have become less noticeable.

Today, Chris is an intelligent, stable and productive adult. He loves books, art, and music. You could never tell he had ever had such an accident, unless you noticed the huge scar on his head where the left side of his skull had been removed during surgery.

Our family would not have survived this time without the Lord, our faith and our friends. The love and presence of all of them brought us through this awful time. We believe that faith, family, and friends can not only witness a great miracle, they can be a part of it.

~Bette Haywood Matero

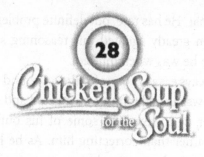

28

Don't Give Up...

Perseverance is the hard work you do after you get tired of doing the hard work you already did.

~Newt Gingrich

Last year I was nearly killed in a car crash. I spent three months in a coma, followed by a full year and a half in a wheelchair. Now I use a walker. I still go to therapy five days a week. Progress is slow but the important point is that I am still making progress.

I had run fifteen miles just an hour before the wreck. So now my goal is to run marathons again. I'm not nearly there yet, but having a goal is important to my recovery. As unclear as my future may be, I choose to focus not on what I *can't* do because of my TBI but what I *can* do in spite of it. I may not be back yet, but I'm trying!

So to those of you who are facing physical, mental and emotional trials, whether it is TBI or any other challenge, I offer some words of encouragement and lessons I have learned along the way:

Celebrate each small victory.

For me, despite all of my physical challenges, I am now able to write again. That is certainly something to celebrate! It also helps me to express myself and hopefully help others with my words. I put together an anthology with Press 53 about people overcoming adversity. It is called *What Doesn't Kill You.* I wrote a nonfiction short story for it called "Times I Nearly Died." When the book was published, that was another reason to celebrate!

Maintain overall fitness in whatever way you can.

I get up every day and do a set of fifty push-ups and fifty sit-ups. Set a goal and focus your energies on working toward it. Mine is to run marathons. I am very lucky to have a great personal trainer. He comes three times a week and helps my body re-learn to move in ways that allow for walking and balance. Sometimes we work from home. Sometimes we go to the gym where my trainer works. It really is a breathtaking learning experience to be forced to admit defeat and begin again.

Focus on overall healthy living.

My trainer has helped me put together a healthy diet. We added fish oil, which contains omega 3 fatty acids which we've read can help in brain recovery.

Challenge yourself every day with brain activities.

The brain, anyone's brain, needs stimulation. Otherwise — get ready for boredom and depression! Word games. Crossword puzzles. Anything that gets the synapses firing. For me, this means writing. It gives my brain a workout and clearly is improving my memory. When I first tried to relearn writing, I had so much memory trouble that I could not remember at the end of a given sentence what the beginning had been about. But I've kept at it with great results.

Bring out the dogs: It's good for the soul!

Isolating yourself from others will make things harder, and it's important to identify the supportive individuals in your life. Not that these necessarily have to be human. So... bring out the dogs! Silly as it may sound, it has been a fantastically rewarding part of my process to spend time with pets. Dogs in particular. It would seem that dogs are specifically designed for helping people with memory exercises. Watching as the dog gladly repeats fetching over and over again reminds me of the importance of repetition and perseverance.

Do not become discouraged: Patience!

Hang in there. The worst aspect of this entire ordeal has got to be the unavoidable fact that you have to relearn everything. And so, if there is one piece of advice I would give readily to anyone with a brain injury, it is this: The brain, while fairly elastic, is a complicated machine. Be patient! Patience is an essential component of this sort of recovery. So buckle in; you've got a long, slow road ahead of you, and shortcuts do not exist. Just call your friendly dog over and get ready to wait.

Sit! Stay! Good dog! One day, pup, we'll run a marathon together. You just wait. I am dead set that one day I will run a marathon again. One day.

~Murray Dunlap

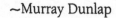

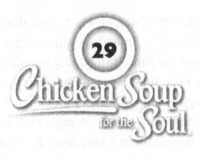

29

A Tougher Course

Green is the prime color of the world and that from which its loveliness arises.
~Pedro Calderón de la Barca

On February 8th, 2012 my ride to work involved a work truck, an ambulance, and an orange helicopter. While driving to my job, I was involved in an accident and instead of going to work I ended up at Sunnybrook Trauma Center. I was informed that I had six broken ribs, a flail chest, a broken collarbone, shattered scapula, fractured vertebrae and a traumatic brain injury.

Once I was discharged from the hospital, much of which I don't remember, life was a lot different and very scary. The world was in such a big hurry and I just happened to slow down. I can't recall all of the adjustments that were made, most of which fell on my spouse Leeann and my family. I know that I slept on the couch for two months because I couldn't walk up the stairs to my bedroom. I couldn't get to the bathroom. My balance and poor vision put me at risk for falls and injuries. I was completely disoriented and couldn't remember where things were in my house or what time of day it was.

I don't remember much of those initial five months, but I do remember the doctor telling me that I might never golf again. That's when physiotherapy and occupational therapy became more important to me. When asked by these professionals what my goals were, I replied, "To prove you all wrong!" I was determined to become just as skilled a golfer as I once was. It was a good thing that I had a left-handed swing because the limited mobility of my right arm would have ended my game for sure. Instead, my mobility improved with a golf club in my hand, a more natural movement I suppose.

I grew up playing golf with my grandfather. I used to putt into his shoes in the living room. I first swung a club at the age of seven and I got my first 9-iron about a year later. As I got older, my game became more aggressive and competitive: my motto was win at all costs! After all, the loser had to buy the beer at the 19th hole. The golf course was my escape from the world's problems.

After eight months of rehabilitation, my occupational therapist suggested that we head out to the driving range. I thought, "Well, it's about time!" But reality set in after I hit four balls. I threw my clubs on the ground and said, "I don't hit the ball like this; let's go home." But since I'm not a quitter, I got back out there with my rehab therapist and friends and learned patience. I hit more balls each time and slowly gained the confidence to play again.

My neuropsychologist introduced me to another brain injury survivor who took me under his wing and taught me a valuable lesson: "Who you were before is not who you are now," he told me. "So play to your ability." I joined a group of gentlemen who all have brain injuries, and we hit the indoor golf simulator once a week. Once summer came, we joined a golf league. Was I the same? No. I had a changed game. In fact I remember one afternoon when the four of us were approached by the golf marshal. He may have thought we were drunk. Little did he know we were just four guys with brain injuries!

I used to play with friends, but now I play my best ball with other survivors. I beat my occupational therapist twice and my rehab support worker. Driving a golf cart had to be approved by the OT. When teeing it up, it now involves one eye closed, balance check and a lot of muscle memory. I have to pay more attention and the result is not as far or as straight. Heck, I don't even know where the ball is going sometimes. Double vision makes the putting game interesting!

I enjoy the game more now than I ever did before. I am slower and less competitive. It's now a form of entertainment, exercise and fun. I take more time to be respectful and patient with others and in turn, others enjoy golfing with me. Golf helps me with my rehabilitation as well because it improves my balance, vision, and concentration. It also helps with my mood and my sleep. Golf keeps me social and it makes me keep my emotions in check. Finally, where the 19th hole was the "beer hole" now it is just the hole for bragging rights.

What does my golf game have to do with my recovery, you may ask? Well, a lot. My game uses all the drive and determination that helped me move forward with my brain injury. I was told that I would never play again and today I can keep up with the best of them. When on the golf course, I have no worries, no pain and no injury. When playing golf, you focus on just hitting that little white ball. I have learned to be patient, to accept my limitations, and to enjoy life, because you never know when it might be taken from you.

What's next for me? Ten years until the senior tour!

~Jay McLaughlin

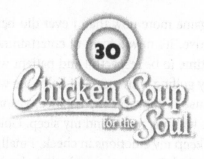

An In-Between Place

There is a bit of insanity in dancing that does everybody a great deal of good.
~Edwin Denby

Ken pulled open the Velcro belt holding him safely in his wheelchair and stood up, shaky yet supporting himself on the parallel bars in the busy rehab gym. I stood in front of him, between the bars. The big windows over our shoulders framed the brilliant blue sky over the Catalina Mountains outside Tucson, their brown flanks dotted with cacti and spindly desert trees. It was a beautiful January day, but I was too preoccupied to enjoy it.

"Sweetie, you know what to do," I said, even though I wasn't sure he did. His short-term memory was badly damaged, and he didn't remember anything from ten minutes ago, let alone yesterday. "You've done this plenty of times before. Hold onto the bars and walk forward."

My husband pointed his face at me and smiled, but his gaze was focused somewhere in the distance, as it had been since a hit-and-run driver left him with a traumatic brain injury a few weeks earlier. Now he was trapped inside his injured brain. The damage was invisible to imaging scans, but his behavior revealed the truth of what had happened to him. Present but not present, Ken existed in some in-between place.

"Okay," he said and began shuffling forward. He was very wobbly on his feet. The TBI had compromised his balance and his ability to walk in a straight line.

I came to the rehab hospital every morning and stayed until after Ken ate dinner. His therapists knew me by now and allowed me to assist with his treatment. Being of use to my husband helped me, too, temporarily easing the near-constant panic that had welled up as soon as I learned about his accident.

We had been married exactly nine months before what we came to call the "brain wreck." I tried not to let myself think of what the future might hold for us, now that my husband had been violently altered by the collision caused by the never-identified white sedan. Instead, I focused on putting one foot in front of the other, just as Ken was doing between the parallel bars, pushing myself through each grueling day.

In the first days after the accident, when Ken was in the ICU, he was often delirious and agitated, thrashing and calling out words no one could understand. Yet he grew calmer whenever he knew I was there. He seemed to recognize that I was important to him, even if he didn't know why or who I was. Each week, he improved incrementally, but he existed in some inward place, unable at least for now to overcome the damage to his frontal lobes and elsewhere in his brain. His speech was lively, even though he often made no sense due to fluent aphasia, but he could not connect in any meaningful way with anyone. Not even me.

After being admitted to the rehab hospital, he began calling me "Boo," from out of nowhere. One day in his room, I asked, "Ken, what's my name?"

A haunted look came over his face as he struggled to remember. He looked as if he might cry.

"Oh, sweetie! It's okay," I reassured him, taking his hand. "My name is Barbara. You just forgot for a while."

"Barbara," he repeated. "Good. That's a good name."

Curious to see what else he had forgotten, I asked, "Who am I?"

The haunted look returned. "Um, a nurse?" he asked.

I made myself smile. "No, silly. I'm your wife. My name is Barbara and I'm your wife."

Ken grinned in my direction, looking past my shoulder. "Okay."

Ten minutes later, he had forgotten again, so his speech therapist hung a sign near his bed that said, "My wife's name is Barbara." We weren't sure he could read or comprehend it.

Not yet understanding what brain injury could do to a person, I grew impatient with his lack of connection. Often I held his hand or stroked his forehead or hugged him, yet he made no move towards me. We were newlyweds, for God's sake! Couldn't he at least reach out to me a little bit? According to the nurses, Ken asked every evening where I was and when I would be back. My dear husband could not remember my goodbye kiss and promise to return the next morning—or that I had been there at all. It appeared he wanted me nearby, but even as we stood there in the gym, the chasm between us felt impossible to bridge.

As Ken walked toward me between the parallel bars, I encouraged him to keep going. He reached the end, so we turned around the other way. Several times, we repeated the trip. We faced the big, sun-filled windows and stood side by side, holding on to the bar to do leg lifts, squats, and a few other basic exercises to help Ken regain his strength.

"You're getting stronger every day," I told him. "You won't need that chair much longer, I bet."

"Yeah. I'm going to get better," he said. He had uttered these words many times, even though he could not possibly know the effort that would be required of him and how long it would take. Doubtful, I nevertheless prayed he was right.

During those horrible days, I existed in my own in-between place. I was Ken's wife, but would I now mainly be his caregiver? For how long? Could someone really recover from a brain injury as bad as his? What if he couldn't go back to work? Would we have a future together? What if I eventually discovered I couldn't live with him any longer because it was too hard? Would I stay out of guilt? Did I need to sacrifice myself for him? Already, I was exhausted. Terror and panic felt like the only emotions I had ever experienced—secondary traumatic stress, a counselor would later call it. How long could I keep going?

Ken walked out from between the bars. I followed. He turned toward me and held out his arms—the first time since the accident—and pulled me close as he hummed a tune in my ear. We began simply rocking from foot to foot. Tears filled my eyes at this tender gesture. We had often done this at home before the wreck, spontaneously grabbing one another for a few minutes of slow dancing as one of us hummed a made-up tune.

The sounds of the noisy gym receded as Ken's arms enveloped me. Everyone else in the room seemed to vanish. For the first time, I felt hope rising—for his recovery, for our future.

"Thank you for helping me, Boo," Ken whispered into my hair. "I'm working hard to get better for you."

Amazed at his words, I looked into his eyes, which still gazed into the distance, then snuggled back into his shoulder, grateful for this sign of recognition.

Ken eventually remembered my name. Forty long days after the brain wreck, he came home and, slowly, we recovered together. Ten years later, he still calls me "Boo" on purpose, because he knows I love it.

~Barbara Stahura, CJF

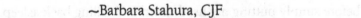

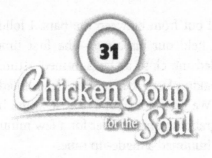

Not Just a Run

There are only two mistakes one can make along the road to truth:
not going all the way and not starting.
~Buddha

Suddenly I awoke. I saw my sister Melinda sitting beside me staring. "Aren't I supposed to be at work?" I asked her.

"No John, you have today off," she answered.

I noticed I was in a hospital gown, tied to a hospital bed. "Melinda, why can't I move my left leg?"

"John, you were in a car accident." I fell silent for a moment or so, before simply putting my head down and falling back asleep.

Over the next little bit, I learned that I had suffered a catastrophic traumatic brain injury in a car accident on my way to work almost two weeks before. My legs hadn't been hurt or damaged by the accident. My brain had simply forgotten how to operate my left side. I began the usual rehabilitation that TBI survivors must deal with, including physical therapy and cognitive techniques.

Friends and family flocked to my side, offering support, aid, advice, and just wanting to see me. As is extremely common amongst people dealing with TBI, I developed anxiety, depression, along with dealing with all the emotional problems that come with the entire situation.

It was so frightening to have to rely on a chair with wheels attached to get anywhere. The idea of going down the hall to watch

TV was daunting due to the effort required; I kept traveling in circles around the hallways.

One of the things I immediately noticed was how much the gym calmed me. Growing up, I had never been a very physical person. Now I loved it. As the ability to get out of the wheelchair came back, I had to work on my balance and coordination the most. I felt so proud and happy when I finally "graduated" from the chair to a walker, then the walker to a cane; eventually I was able to stand and walk unaided. Throughout all of this time and to this day I still can't put on my shoes without sitting down, and likely never will; but at least I am able to walk.

The gym provided the opportunity to use exercise bikes, elliptical machines, a treadmill and a track. I loved using these facilities, laying the groundwork for what was to unfold almost two years after the accident, when my close friend Rick, who is a runner, persuaded me to try it. At first it was very frustrating, as it highlighted and exaggerated all of my deficits. I started to learn more about what my recovery would entail. I was making gains physically, but now had to manage the barriers of cognitive fatigue, and lack of initiative and follow through, all of which make achieving goals very hard.

After running regularly for a month or so though, I started to love every second of it. The constant chatter in my mind quieted down. I had such a serene feeling when I was done. I even got a chip to put into my shoe to track my performance with my smartphone, which provided the ability to follow my running distances and times, giving me something solid to mark my progress, as well as giving me the push to keep going.

As the months went on, I started running farther and faster. Rick decided it would be a good idea to challenge me to run a half marathon with him. At first I was extremely reluctant. But I finally decided to accept the challenge and began looking into training options. I had only been seriously running for about two and a half months and had only participated in one organized run, a 3K.

As time went on, and the date of the race drew nearer, Rick hurt his knee. He was very apologetic that he would not be able to run with me, however very insistent that I still run it on my own. Obviously I felt heartbroken and upset. My best friend who had made me a runner wouldn't be running my biggest race with me.

September 22, 2013, race day, was upon me. At this point in time, it had only been two and a half years since I woke in that hospital bed, and nine months and 631 kilometers since beginning to run. I sat down, nervously shaking, put my shoes on, and proceeded to run my first half marathon. There is no way to accurately describe the feeling of slapping the headphones on, and after a while, realizing how much ground I was covering. I was doing it. I was running a half marathon. I had initiated something and followed through with it. I was accomplishing my goal.

My time ended up being 1:59:25, a time seasoned runners would be proud of. I felt so overwhelmed at the finish line, I almost started crying. I felt so silly. Why would I feel that emotional about putting one foot in front of the other rapidly and repeatedly? Then I realized it was seeing the culmination of months of research and work unfolding into something satisfying, a monumental accomplishment, not just for my physical side, but my cognitive and emotional sides as well. Crossing the finish line wasn't just running a race; it was organized executive function at work.

Through several group therapy sessions, and other means, I have connected with a few people with TBI, all of whom also have to sit down to put on shoes. I realize however, that almost all people who have suffered TBI need to use many aids, strategies and alternate techniques to achieve their goals. One other thing I have learned is that when those things are used, whether it be a date book for daily routine, or sitting down to strap on footwear, watch out. There is no telling how far any of us TBI survivors will go. The road to recovery is yours to travel down as you will.

~Johnkle

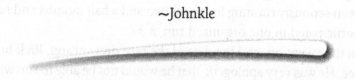

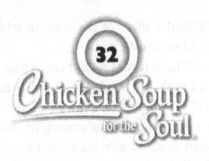

The Making of a Miracle

What lies behind us and what lies before us are tiny matters,
compared to what lies within us.

~Ralph Waldo Emerson

It's October 6, 2002, one of those autumn days when the air smells of dried leaves and the trees are pumpkin-colored. I'm at work when I hear my cell phone buzz under my desk. It stops. Then buzzes again. It's my daughter Annie. She's sobbing.

"Mom, Casey was in a motorcycle accident. They had to cut away part of his skull. You've got to get to Charleston. He's at the Medical University of South Carolina. Hurry, Mom. Hurry." I cup a hand over my mouth to muffle animal cries rising from the depths of me.

The drive to Charleston usually takes three hours. Not today. Annie is waiting for me, her eyes red and swollen. We rush down the hallway into the intensive care unit. Casey's skull, swathed in gauze, bulges on one side. His nose is widened. Lips puffed. I can barely discern this face as my son's. My nineteen-year-old boy. Behind me, I hear the sound of a nurse's rubber-soled shoes squeak on the tile floor.

"Your son was on his motorcycle when he was hit by a car," she says, her tone low and soft. "The ambulance got to him just minutes after an anonymous 911 call came in. We don't know how long he was lying there."

I hear her, but I barely absorb what she is saying.

"The impact to Casey's skull caused his brain to swell. The

neurosurgeon removed a piece of the bone to release pressure. He saw a blood clot and suctioned it out."

I want to ask, "Is he in pain? Can he hear us if we talk to him? Is he going to live?" But I can't. My words get stuck. My body grows numb. I feel like my world is wobbling on a three-legged chair. I pray.

Twenty-four hours later, the neurosurgeon has put Casey into a medically induced coma to give his brain time to heal. Machines beep and blink. I talk to my son.

"Casey, I just want you to know that I'm not going to give up on you. I am going to pull the low hanging fruit from every spiritual tree — call on God and every one of His angels to heal you. I promise to leave no stone unturned. Do you hear me, son?"

One day slips into another. Casey is unchanged. The neurologists fight to minimize the effects of the trauma to his brain, fight to save his life. I place my hopes on less traditional methods of wellness. I hold onto a mustard seed, spritz my boy with Lourdes holy water, use alternative healing techniques on him, and even summon the Blessed Mother Mary and her angels with prayers.

In time, time measured in the agony of minutes, hours, days, nights and weeks, Casey improves. Physically. That is when the real challenges begin.

On the step-down hospital floor, and in a rehab center, Casey struggles to speak, to walk, and even to eat again on his own. Watching him tugs at my heartstrings.

His time in rehab comes to an end. The shell of my boy walks through the door of our house, yet it appears a total stranger is living inside, another challenge to understand.

I must find a new way to parent my son, to meet this challenge head-on, to overcome this obstacle. The days grind on. I visit a spiritualist church for strength, hope, guidance, anything. I pester Casey's kind doctor for answers. He describes in plain English what frontal lobe damage is and details the repercussions of a traumatic brain injury. I take notes.

"The frontal lobe handles planning and organizing," he tells me. "It also plays an important role in managing emotions—dealing with hunger, aggression and sexual drive. Separate sections of the brain control those primitive emotions, and they're equipped with a 'stop' button that prevents people from doing something inappropriate. The slightest thing—something someone says or does, a loud noise, a scream—can send Casey into overload. Before you know it, he acts out."

"What can I do to help?" I ask.

"The best tool is a time-out. Let's say Casey is so angry he wants to throw something. Get him out of the environment or away from the person who's angering him. Have him go for a walk or sit in a different room with a door closed. Whatever works best." I sigh. Easier said than done.

Recovery has been a winding road filled with potholes, but four years after the accident that nearly took his life, Casey received his associate's degree from Trident Technical College. In that moment, that wondrous moment, I realized that sometimes we don't know what God knows. According to Casey's doctors, in the majority of traumatic brain injury cases the patient shows the most change in the first two years. But by the grace of God, Casey continued to improve far beyond that deadline.

Nine years after my son suffered a traumatic brain injury, I am finally able to let go of two fears—never seeing him get married—and not getting to dance at his wedding. Casey proposed to Lyly and they were married at Carothers Coastal Gardens—an enchanting Spanish-heritage home filled with lush gardens, overlooking Galveston Bay. With twinkling eyes and a glowing smile, Casey stretches out his hand and draws me close, and we dance on a dime. I'm caught up in the miracle... the dance of my lifetime... this dance with my son... my precious, precious son. He's not only walking... and talking... he's dancing... we're dancing.

What helped Casey turn the corner? What allowed him to have another chance at life? Was it the constant care of doctors and nurses? The power of prayer that circled the globe? His family's undying love and support? My abiding faith, hope and perseverance?

Maybe it was all of the above.

~Pattie Welek Hall

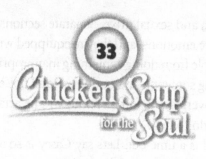

Joanie

Our greatest glory is not in never falling, but in rising every time we fall.
~Confucius

"Larry, I'm hurt," Joanie yelled, as I jogged around the corner some distance behind her. I raced toward where she was lying to see blood dripping down her face. My first thought was that she had been struck by a car and tossed onto the lawn where she lay—that's how torn and battered she appeared.

"My feet got caught in my sneaker laces, and I fell on my face onto the asphalt. I crawled over here to get out of the road. I felt such a whack when I hit," she said, adding, "this can't be good."

It wasn't. The emergency room physician concluded that she had sustained a subdural hematoma. In an instant, my wife of almost four decades went from being a vibrant, physically fit woman enjoying the prime of her life, to someone seriously injured with a traumatic brain injury. In the following days, Joanie experienced extreme head pain, confusion, lethargy, nausea, sleep disturbances, impaired attention, memory loss, a speech disorder, hearing deficits, emotional distress and behavior changes. Within ten days of that freak fall, she could not respond, move, stand, or walk. Within a month, she experienced three emergency room visits, two hospitalizations, and one brain surgery.

At home after her first hospitalization, Joanie's symptoms—especially her head pain—began to worsen as fluid accumulated around her brain. I found her in bed a few mornings later unable to respond, walk, or talk. I called an ambulance to take her back to the hospital.

Days into that second hospitalization, the neurosurgeon took my grown daughter Janna and me aside to tell us, "She's going to need surgery to drain the fluid; I've scheduled the operation for seven thirty tomorrow morning."

Just after arriving home that same night, I received a phone call from another member of the neurosurgery team saying that the swelling in her cranium had increased suddenly. "We're not going to wait until tomorrow morning to operate," he said. "We're going to perform the surgery at eleven o'clock tonight." Janna and I hurried back to the hospital, arriving just in time to see the surgical team wheeling my wife into the operating room. As they did, I barely managed to choke out, "Take good care of my girl."

At one o'clock in the morning, the neurosurgeon came to the hushed waiting room to tell us the results. "The surgery went well," he said. "Her breathing tube is even out."

At that point, both Janna and I breathed a lot easier ourselves. We stayed with Joanie every day in the hospital, saddened to see the stitches along the nine-inch incision on her shaved scalp, listening to the quiet shush-click of the inflatable cuffs on her legs designed to help prevent blood clots.

While her symptoms began to lessen after surgery, Joanie still had a long rehabilitation to go through to regain the physical, cognitive, and coordination abilities her injury had impaired. After her discharge, a rehabilitation team of four therapists made regular home visits over several months. They worked on rebuilding her core strength and balance, restoring the planning and sequencing abilities that normal living requires, and returning her reading, speech, and memory to their former levels. Then it was several more months of outpatient speech and reading therapy to continue strengthening her cognitive functioning. Joanie vigorously and conscientiously practiced all the exercises her therapists gave her. She was highly motivated to get better. Janna and I (and our son, Todd, who had flown in from the opposite coast) saw it as our jobs to be her cheerleaders, listening posts, and confidence builders as she worked hard to regain function.

Still, it took almost a year after her descent into helplessness for her to fight her way fully back to health. In this, she was aided by the love and support not only of our family but also our friends who plied us with visits, cards, food, and concern, and the talented health care providers and rehabilitation therapists who treated her. Remarkably, throughout most of this ordeal, Joanie was conscious and aware of what had happened. The irony of having been injured while exercising to keep in good health didn't escape her, as she repeated often what we came to call her mantra: "What a stupid thing to have happen to me."

One day, late into the year of her rehabilitation, Joanie and I were out walking. As we walked, she asked if I happened to see a segment earlier that week on one of the national morning television shows where people were invited to summarize their lives in just three words and to write those three words on their hands. I said I hadn't seen it. Joanie introduced it to me by commenting how deeply emotional it was for her. She said it showed people expressing highly charged sentiments, like "Miss my soldier" and "I love life."

She went on, "The one that sticks in my mind was..." but she couldn't finish her sentence. Her eyes welling up, she said, "I don't know if I can get this out." We fell into a long silence and continued to walk as she regained her composure. After several minutes, she took a deep breath and began to speak. As she did, there were no resounding cheers, no triumphant fanfares. Only quiet tears of victory.

"The one I want to tell you about," she said, "was the person who wrote a sentiment on each of her hands. On one hand, it said, 'I FELL DOWN.' On the other hand, it said, 'I GOT UP.'"

~Larry C. Kerpelman, Ph.D

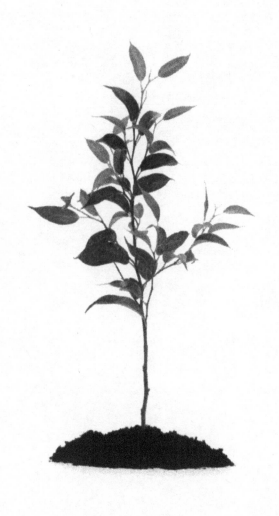

Recovering *from* Traumatic Brain Injuries

Healing Power of Mother Nature

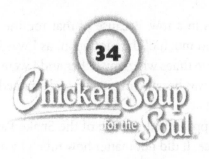

34

Reaching for the Sky

One may walk over the highest mountain one step at a time.
~Barbara Walters

I t was so difficult. We inched our way up, climbing the Snake Path of Masada, a fortress in the mountains of ancient Israel where the Jewish people held off the Roman emperor's army for three years. As in the days of Masada, my trip up the Snake Path was arduous. However, I kept reminding myself as I ascended with my father, "The easy things in life are usually not worth doing."

I had learned that lesson the hard way. I had been shot in the head at the young age of nineteen, causing a traumatic brain injury. I did survive with much help and determination. Some say I have turned surviving into thriving, but I just try. I have disabilities as a result of the injury; however, I believe that all human beings have their own challenges and disabilities.

I kept repeating that statement to myself as I attempted to climb the steep mountain. There were many places on the path where there was not enough room for both my father (who was holding me tightly) and me to climb side by side. My father, therefore, held me perhaps even tighter as he followed me slowly up the path.

As we climbed higher and higher, I was also remembering how difficult it had been to train for this climb. Months before, my father and I would climb the twenty-five flights of stairs at St. Luke's Episcopal Hospital in Houston. At the end of several months of training we had reached the point where we were climbing the hospital stairs three times in a row. Because of that routine, I was breathing easily as I climbed much of the mountain, as I was basically in good shape. (There were times when my father and I were having difficulty breathing, but it was because of tension and strained nerves, not lack of conditioning.)

But as we approached the top of the Snake Path a broad smile came over my face. It did not matter how much I was hurting; also, it did not matter that we were thousands of miles away from our home in Houston. Actually, for a brief moment in time nothing seemed to matter at all, except that I was accomplishing my goal—climbing the steep fortress of Masada.

Just then, as I was twenty steps from the summit, I heard a group of Israeli soldiers at the top of Masada all applauding my achievement. I was so proud, not because I had climbed Masada and not because Israeli soldiers had applauded my accomplishment, but because I had achieved my goal.

Everyone in life has his own mountains to climb, some big, some small—but mountains nonetheless. I believe the important thing in a person's life is trying to overcome one's obstacles. I thought about that as I reached the very top of Masada—and then I collapsed for a few minutes. Lying with my face on the ground I thought: "I did it. I did it." But I quickly realized that I had many more and different goals still to reach. I smiled and thought, "Which one is next?"

~Michael Jordan Segal, MSW

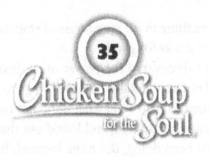

35

Taming the Hurricane

*I can't change the direction of the wind, but I can adjust my sails
to always reach my destination.*
~Jimmy Dean

It was like a bomb had gone off. There was nothing much left to the home I shared with my wife and kids in a Southern Florida county. It was gone. Just gone. Hurricane Andrew took not only my home, it also took the peace I'd managed to tenuously keep for years since my severe traumatic brain injury.

I'd found an employer who understood my issues and allowed me to work in and organize my own space, also be solitary and take breaks when I needed them. My wife seemed to have accepted my behavioral quirks and would tell our children, "Don't mind him—you know how your father is." Things were status quo and were moving along as well as I and most of my friends and family could imagine.

But then there was the storm. And our home was gone.

We had insurance and could rebuild. We hadn't lost anyone we loved. There was much to be thankful for, but the storm had planted its own eye in my mind, and like Andrew itself, it was slow to start but building in intensity.

I hadn't lost everything, and I knew it on one level, but my brain couldn't comprehend the overwhelming change and big picture. The wider the picture got, the wilder my brain swirled. I began to cry uncontrollably every day. It seemed gone. All gone. We could rebuild the house but something in my own house of emotional cards seemed shattered. I feared it was for good.

That's when I discovered the power of meditation and support groups. It started out accidentally. For relief I'd go to a quiet room and "Zen out." It seemed to help somewhat although the peace wouldn't last for long. I began researching and found out that meditation was similar to what I'd been doing, but more focused. It could build neural pathways and allow the brain to rest, rebuild, and stay focused on the present moment.

There are many ways to meditate. I tried going to a Buddhist retreat to practice, but it was hard to stay focused on that place between breathing in and breathing out; focus is hard for me with my TBI. I could see the potential though. I knew I couldn't give up. Giving up is easy, but it's the most important impulse to fight.

I found a place called Centerpointe. It offered a program that not only allowed me to meditate more deeply than traditional meditation methods but also to experience the benefits of meditation quickly, which is what I really needed. I found success with their approach thanks to the dual scientific and spiritual focus. When I put on the headphones, the first feeling I have is immense relief. There are no problems in that place. In fact, at times there are euphoric feelings that last all day.

I've actually had people ask me, why formal meditation? Why not just go into the room like I did before and take some moments of peace? I found there is a difference between the two. There is a calming structure, a discipline that helps me function emotionally and also helps my brain develop other neural pathways to deal more effectively when faced with skills I need but had lost due to the TBI. It's planned relief rather than feeling you have to run away and isolate yourself.

Like the accident that changed my life and brain forever, I can't say I'm glad Hurricane Andrew happened, but I can say that what seemed like another misfortune led me to something I needed so that I could be the most whole I could be. Although the winds of life will always swirl, I've found how I can tame the hurricane.

~Pete Daigle

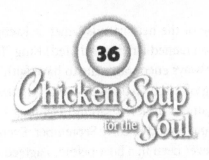

36

Uncharted Waters

Only those who will risk going too far can possibly find out how far one can go.

~T.S. Eliot

After graduating from college in May of 2006, I planned to start a promising career, get a nice car, find my future wife, buy a house, and maybe even have a kid. It seemed to be the normal path for a twenty-three-year-old college graduate from a great family with plenty of opportunity ahead.

I interviewed for multiple jobs and received a couple of offers, but I was in no hurry for my post-graduation celebratory lifestyle to end. On July 4th I drove drunk after a party. Didn't I know it was dangerous and criminal to drink and drive? Yes.

My parents got that dreaded early morning phone call. "Your son has serious head trauma," said the voice. Five weeks unresponsive in the ICU followed by six weeks of intensive inpatient therapy all led up to a year of a neuro-rehab program. Believe it or not, then came the hard part.

I tried so hard, and at times still do, to get back to being the kid I was before or to become the man I planned to be. I still play golf and work out, but it's not the way it used to be. It's been frustratingly tough to accept diminished abilities at doing things I used to do with ease. My anger and depression grew. It was at the Krempels Center, a community-based day program for brain injury survivors, in Portsmouth, New Hampshire where I began a new life. New friends, additional support, and the realization that I was not alone meant the world to me. One of the new friends I met at Krempels is a retired orthopedic surgeon named Dr. Edward (Ted) King. Ted has become a great friend and always encourages me to have faith and do my best.

In the spring of 2010, Ted asked me if I'd crew for him in the Robie Pierce Regatta, a disabled sailing regatta at Larchmont Yacht Club on Long Island Sound in early September. Even though I wasn't a sailor, having never been in a boat before, I agreed. I was always an anxious kid and after my accident my anxiety intensified. I usually can't figure out the root cause of the constant worry and fear I feel. Maybe the impending doom that follows me around is worry about another car accident. But without memory of the traumatic event, I can't process the ambiguous distressing thoughts I have. I had developed some unhealthy coping mechanisms by this time, one of which was to cancel plans or not follow through on commitments, thinking it would bring me relief.

The night before I was to leave for Larchmont, New York, I felt intense fear and left Ted a message saying I wasn't going to the race. Shortly thereafter I received a phone call from Bill Sandberg, who told me not to worry and that the point of the whole regatta was to have fun. There were no expectations. Bill was the AB (able-bodied sailor) in our three-man crew. The AB is the person who takes over in the event of an emergency and completes the actions the disabled sailors can't physically carry out. He's a great guy and his humor put me at ease.

I went to the regatta, even winning my first-ever race, a practice race, with Bill joking, "You should quit while you're ahead; it can only be downhill from first place." We came in fourth out of eighteen boats that weekend. Being part of a team and involved in competitive sports again was thrilling. The confidence I gained in facing my fears, real or imagined, continues to help me as I face new challenges. Since that first race, Ted and I have competed in five additional regattas with quite a bit of success. With Bill, we even won the 2011 National Championship in the development class. In fact, just this past weekend we raced in the championship class of the 2013 US Sailing National Championship in Milwaukee with AB

Dan Rugg, winning the final race and placing second overall in the championship division.

Finding a challenge that I never would have attempted prior to my TBI and completing it with unexpected success and enjoyment has built my confidence. Sailing is something I'm proud of post-brain injury. When sailing, I don't think about the way it used to be, because I never sailed before. Racing sailboats is completely uncharted waters for me and that is one of the reasons I've grown to love it.

~Jim Scott

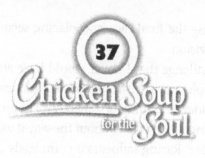

Jared's Fishing Logs

Efforts and courage are not enough without purpose and direction.
~John F. Kennedy

It had been five days since our seventeen-year-old son, Jared, had been ejected from a crashing car and sustained a traumatic brain injury. He lay in a coma surrounded by whirring machines, wires, and worry.

My husband Rich, our older son Cole, and I kept watch at Jared's bedside, praying of course, for a miracle. Doctors cautioned us not to research TBI on the Internet, explaining that the range of TBIs was enormous and we would just have to wait patiently to learn the extent of Jared's injury. Still, nobody could promise that he would wake up, walk, or talk again.

It was early July and just a week before Jared had had an enviable summer ahead of him. A high school senior, he was looking forward to long, carefree days on the lake. He was a familiar fixture there, greeting every sunrise with a fishing pole in one hand and a tackle box in the other. We longed for a glimpse of that boy and logged into his computer, searching for his voice.

There we found his fishing logs.

The purpose of a fishing log is to save pertinent information that can be reviewed later to remember the what, when, where, why, and how of each fishing excursion. Jared's logs featured meticulous detail about weather conditions, moon phase, water conditions, locations, lures and times. They were a testament to the hundreds of hours

Jared spent out on his twelve-foot boat, and to his innate discipline and patience while waiting to make a catch.

Rich liked to say that fishing was in Jared's blood; it's what made him tick. The two of them had been fishing together since Jared was eight years old, either at the ninety-five acre lake down the street from our house, or out on the Cape Cod Canal.

Initially, reading his fishing logs made us cry. The thought that Jared might not fish again was gut wrenching. But we vowed to take one day at a time and took to reading excerpts of the logs out loud. We believed Jared could hear us and knew that nothing would be more interesting to him than accounts of his own fishing escapades.

Miraculously, Jared came out of the coma. His TBI was severe enough that he needed to re-learn the basic tasks of daily living and enter a long-term rehabilitation center.

Toward the end of his eighty-nine day stay in rehab, we were allowed to bring Jared home for daytime weekend visits. On the first of these visits I asked Jared, "If you could choose to do anything you wanted today, what would it be?"

Without hesitation, he answered, "Go fishing."

So, off to the lake father and son went, just like old times. It wasn't a movie ending—they didn't come back with a catch for that night's dinner—but they did come back triumphant. In Rich's words, "I knew that day that fishing was the one thing in Jared's life that remained true. The passion was still there, making him tick."

It took enormous effort for Jared to concentrate on his return to fishing and sometimes it was exhausting. At the time, he wasn't even thinking about his fishing logs. So Rich would come home and make notes about each trip—mainly, the what, when, where, why, and how of Jared's progress. It became a way for Rich to participate in Jared's rehab, making him, and us, feel a little less helpless.

Rich's entry, on that first day back to the lake noted that it was a cold autumn day, the sun was shining and the New England foliage seemed extra bright. He explained that Jared struggled, that he couldn't get his hands and fingers to do what he wanted, but he kept trying. Casting, reeling, over and over; he just wouldn't give up.

Soon the fishing logs took on new meaning and became a source of comfort for all of us. Rich felt productive keeping a fishing journal for Jared, and Cole and I eagerly read each entry. Documenting Jared's rehabilitation through the logs was therapeutic. Later, Jared would read his dad's entries and marvel at the story of determination and progress they told.

As a result of his TBI, Jared suffers from short-term memory loss and has trouble organizing thoughts and processing verbal information. But he's reached tremendous milestones thanks to a support system of family and friends, community, and dedicated professionals.

We think the real miracle is that Jared spent years honing his fishing logs, and it turned out to be the preparation he needed for dealing with his TBI. Today, Jared relies on checklists, mostly maintained on his iPhone, to get through each day. Checklists are critical to his success. They help him remember the what, when, where, why, and how. We have no doubt that Jared's practice keeping detailed fishing logs before his accident is the reason he is so adept and comfortable with using checklists today.

There was a time when Jared's fishing logs made us cry. Then they became a lifeline, linking us to his rehabilitation. Now we celebrate that Jared's passion and instinct for creating a great fishing experience has come full circle.

~Janine L. Osburn

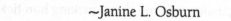

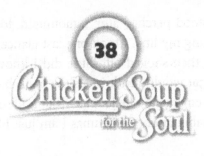

38

The Nature of My Motivation

Look deep into nature and then you will understand everything better.
~Albert Einstein

I snap on my helmet, pull down my goggles, strap my foot to my board, take a deep breath, and look around. This is one of my very favorite moments. The perfectly blue sky rolls out endlessly before me in all directions. It is dotted here and there with the most beautiful fluffy clouds. What mesmerizes me the most is the simple lack of rhyme or reason to their placement. They are just wherever they happen to be peacefully floating, wherever they fit—no questions asked and no reason to rearrange. As I observe and relax and take in their all-encompassing beauty, I find myself in a wonderful state, pure bliss. If we all started our day with a simple, heart-opening cloud meditation, maybe we would all be in such a state.

As the clouds part, endless peaks reaching to the heavens and beyond are revealed. They are so expansive that I have to stare and stare until my eyes can pick out the many layers in the blue sky. It is mesmerizing. It's as if the clouds were majestically placed beside each other. Now the entire horizon is a spread of stately peaks against an endless horizon.

I have been a skier and snowboarder since the seventh grade. I love the sense of freedom that comes with cruising down the mountain. But I almost wasn't here to enjoy this perfect winter day. Earlier in the season, I stood perched atop a mountain, looking down that last run and picking my line. I took one last glance at the breathtaking horizon, and then shoved off. Little did I know I would take a fall on that run that would result in a slow brain bleed and swelling that required an emergency helicopter ride, a life-saving operation, and weeks of rehabilitation. Sometimes I am just blown away that I am still alive.

What I relied on throughout my recovery was my love of Mother Nature and my desire to return to the sport I hold dear. The same adrenaline that pushed me to ski fast and hard down tall mountains also pushed me to work hard to regain the balance and coordination I would need to return to them.

Standing again on the mountain I love, I find myself wondering if I would take that last run again, knowing what it would lead to. I reflect on the challenges my TBI has caused for myself, my family, and my friends. If I could have a redo, I *should* say no to that run (though I have learned the painful fact that we cannot turn back the hands of time). But we can keep tapping into the strength within. How lucky I am. I take one very deep breath and inhale the winter air of this landscape and reflect on the feeling that comes with this experience. I smile to myself again. I give myself an inward hug and congratulate myself for taking the time to drink in this beauty.

I treasure that sense of freedom that comes when the freshest air in the world is gently brushing your cheeks and you start cruising towards that endless blue sky and her magical clouds. You hear Mother Nature's soft secret whisper as you slowly start your decent. Swish! Swish! This is what I truly believe saved me and helped me get to where I am today. I am grateful as always to Mother Nature. She is such a wonderful gift to us all. She feeds me.

~Robin Lee Rice Whittaker

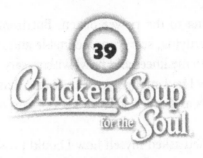

39

Finding Hidden Messages of Hope

Every flower is a soul blossoming in nature.
~Gérard de Nerval

Walking out of the hall to the moonlit forecourt I cradled the magnificent bouquet of flowers in my arms. Applause from the audience was still echoing in my head. What an enchanting evening it had been. As a past teacher at the school, I had been honored to be the guest speaker at the gala dinner to celebrate its 110th anniversary. I inhaled the perfume of the spring flowers—how wonderful it was to be alive!

Just a couple of hours before, when I'd entered this splendid hall I'd felt a shiver go down my spine as, out of the corner of my eye, I caught a glimpse of the ghost of me. I heard my silent screams of two decades before, when I'd first entered this hall on my return to school, after a long absence following my horrific car accident.

Back then I was so ashamed, as I shuffled and wobbled my way in the doorway, my walking stick tap tap tapping as I tried to keep my balance, my black eye patch helping me cope with the swirling mad double world I inhabited. I was empty, lost, sad and crushed. I had no hope that things would improve in the future—indeed I'd been constantly told by the experts that "there is no cure for brain injury." If you'd asked me to look into the future I would have numbly described a one dimensional, monotonous grey world peopled by grey figures. Boring to the power of ten. But ironically the boring world was also terrifying, scary, unpredictable and threatening. How I'd wanted to fall to my knees and howl with misery at the unfairness of life. Fortunately I had enough sense to realize that this would have made the students and other staff members jump out of their skins with fright!

Back then I had asked myself how I could possibly be a teacher again. My brain felt like it had been sucked out by a cruel monster. My emotions were scrambled like eggs. My students were now like the teacher and I was the pupil. Just now, taking a philosophy class, one pupil had taken the chalk out of my hands and said "I'll write on the board for you, Mrs. D. You know you can't spell anymore!"

What had helped me move from that poor broken creature to the person who had just moved an audience by speaking from the heart? Sitting in the car for the journey home I was enveloped by the perfume of the bouquet and I realized that flowers had played a silent role in this transformation.

Once I had moved from the intensive care unit, my new hospital room became a bower of flowers. On one level I felt ashamed that I had no words to thank people for their kindnesses and thoughtfulness (although I did get the message through to my children to write thank you notes which I "signed" with a scribble). But on a deeper level those flowers became symbols of all the people thinking of me, supporting me and wishing me well. Even though I had no sense of smell, and saw double, these flowers became my nonjudgmental companions in the long pain-filled days.

When I returned home I was astonished to be greeted by a shower of golden daffodils nodding their heads. The bulbs I had planted in a dozen pots the day before my accident were blooming, a reminder that life goes on. I was swamped with sadness that the woman who had planted those bulbs (the old me) was not the same woman who now viewed the golden blooms (the new me), but the miracle that those scruffy brown bulbs could be transformed into beautiful yellow trumpets was proof of the power of nature.

Once the daffodils had faded and I'd removed the bulbs to store for next year, I felt compelled to plant container after container of petunias in the pots. I was a tad confused, as I'd never been so extravagant with seedlings before—and then I realized that these annuals were like lucky charms or talismans to show me that one day I, too, just might flower into my old self.

Then came the time when my husband Ted said we should get away for a couple of days. I agreed. I was petrified to be in an automobile as we drove to a favorite seaside town. When we arrived at the cottage, he helped me out of the car and left me resting on the bed while he disappeared. He returned proudly carrying ten tulips in a borrowed vase. Just before the accident we'd been in New York State, and Ted had presented me with ten pink tulips in an empty milk carton. Same flowers, same message, different country, different container. Weeping, I removed my soggy eye patch, and now, with my double vision, there were twice as many tulips, twice the sentiment and twice the gratitude.

Seasons have come and gone, my flowering has continued from my first tentative steps to the letterbox, to returning to school, where I surprised not only myself but also the school manager, by continuing to teaching part-time for a dozen years. Taking philosophy workshops, I encouraged my students to grow new thoughts. At times I could picture their ideas like beautiful flowers spiraling up from their heads. My ideas flowered into my books *Doing Up Buttons* and *Chasing Ideas*, and into creating engaging talks to help people understand their own brain injury experience.

Time passed and I hoped that the fertile soil of my experience, watered by my tears, could produce another flower. At the age of sixty-three, in spite of my double vision, constant pain and memory problems, I embarked on an endeavor to try to discover ways to help brain-injured people make the best of living with brain injury. That is now behind me. My Ph.D is complete. As people with brain injury talked about their experience I was stunned when several participants expressed similar epiphanies: brain injury was both the worst and the best thing that had happened to them. They now appreciate being alive. They are aware of their strengths and their weaknesses and they now feel wise.

As Madeline put it: "Actually it was a flower that told me one day that the world is really worth being in. It was a memorable experience because I was walking around the side of my house and the world had been grey for a long, long time and I saw a red tulip, the bulb I'd put in a pot, and it had flowered red, and honestly, I stopped in my tracks, and it was like wow, and I'll never forget that, and the world then had colour."

When we see colour and hope in our world we can learn to bloom again.

~Dr. Christine Y. Durham

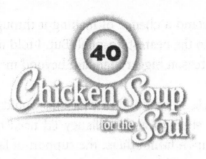

Racing the Sunset

I can be changed by what happens to me. But I refuse to be reduced by it.
~Maya Angelou

L ife, as they say, is what happens when you're busy making other plans. And on July 24, 2004, at the age of twenty-five, life definitely happened. I became the victim and thankful survivor of a near-fatal car accident, leaving me with countless physical wounds and a traumatic brain injury.

A friend and I were doing some sightseeing that hot and sunny Saturday morning, about 1,300 miles from my hometown. En route, I saw a turtle lounging in the middle of the highway. I simply could not leave him there to die, so we pulled over, got out of the car, and my friend picked him up and took him to the other side of the street. And off we went. It was not until ten minutes later that a speeding pick-up truck, with those unnecessarily enormous wheels, came barreling down a side street, ran the stop sign, and plowed into the driver's side of my car, sending us spinning. Upon impact, the driver's side mirror flew into my side window, breaking it, and injuring the left side of my face and my eye, before landing at my friend's feet. Next came the grill of the truck.

My accident was terrifying. Absolutely terrifying. In seconds, everything changed. Had the mirror hit me just an inch higher, I would have been killed instantly. Instead, I lay there, gushing blood from more places than you can count on two hands, in the one hundred degree sun. Given the blood loss, the heat, and the delirium, I didn't think I'd stand a chance of making it through the hour-long ambulance ride to the nearest hospital. But, I told myself, I survived the impact for a reason bigger than and beyond me, and now it was time to fight.

Looking back, I had no idea what that would come to mean. I had no idea the strength and resiliency I'd need to summon from within and rely upon from others; the support of family and friends infused my own. I would see X-rays of screws and plates but it wasn't a piece of electronics I was looking at. It was my face. Having something so foreign in you gets to you after a while. I'd wake up each day not knowing what my eyes would allow me to see—my vision fluctuated so frequently, from complete darkness to doubled, blurred vision, to everything "floating" as if there were no gravity.

There was the constant pain, many medications and surgeries, and the endless doctor and hospital visits. And yet, as other TBI survivors know, all of that is nothing compared to having to face your brain injury on a daily basis. The cognitive fatigue, the sensory overload, the perseveration, the emotional flooding, the confusion, the memory and time lapses, the depression and anxiety, the extreme frustration, and let's not forget those complete "shut-downs." My TBI wreaked a lot of havoc, and stole a lot from me, but over time, I came to realize that it did not touch the essence of who I am; it did not change what I find sacred or precious. What a tremendous and invigorating revelation! Some TBI survivors find the biggest loss to be themselves, but I don't believe that to be true—it's simply a matter of learning to work with the new obstacles and not trying to plow through or will them away.

I learned, much to my chagrin, that my new life would revolve around the sunset—quite literally—as my TBI and vision problems didn't allow me to function well in the dark.

TBI is just that—an injury. An injury that happened to me. It is not me. Remember what used to make you truly happy? Make room for it. The more you are able to bring those things back into your life, the more you will see yourself in you again, and be less apt to let your TBI become your identity.

So what exactly were those plans that this car accident had so rudely interrupted? I was working toward becoming a lawyer, due to begin my third year of law school that September. I was also planning to pursue one of my lifelong dreams of doing Basset Hound rescue work. So, should I abandon my dream of becoming a lawyer, or forge my own path? And how on earth would I do that?

In May 2004, just two months before my car accident, I was listening to a commencement address by a state Supreme Court Justice whom I admired. She said something so striking that resonated with me not only then but also countless times, through every medical hurdle. "You will have your chance to make a difference. The issue is whether you will take it. You can be an ordinary thread in the tunic or you can be that royal touch of purple that gives distinction to the garment. Be that royal touch of purple to the world."

I took the chance and stayed in school. I finished, albeit with a lot of help, and passed two bar exams... on my first try! I forged my own path. I started a legal services non-profit organization with a focus on helping people living with brain injury and educating the general public about TBI. I learned very quickly that to be successful in my work, I needed to control as many variables as I could—given the multitude of limitations I had to manage along with a workload. In short, that meant being my own boss. And so, I found myself becoming an entrepreneur. There's that resiliency at work again.

I have finally been able to truly begin my rescue work. My Basset Hound Kenna was rescued from extreme neglect on Christmas Eve, 2012. Not only has she been fantastic for me—helping to keep some symptoms in check and detecting those overloads before the shut-downs—but she now helps our clients as well. We are quite the dynamic duo; returning veterans and others dealing with PTSD and TBI find the comfort of Kenna coupled with my personal experience compelling, and are much more open about their own struggles. The real kicker? She was rescued just a few miles from my car accident, 1,300 miles away.

Almost ten years later, I still struggle with my TBI. I still have bad and very bad days. I live every day doing my best to balance my own desires with the demands of my injury, and while I don't always win, I do always try.

Once my cognitive fatigue sets in, nothing else will get done until I get recharged. Nothing else positive, that is. As someone who pushes the envelope, it is a daily race to beat the sunset. I live every day racing that sunset, forging my own path.

~Melissa A. Gertz

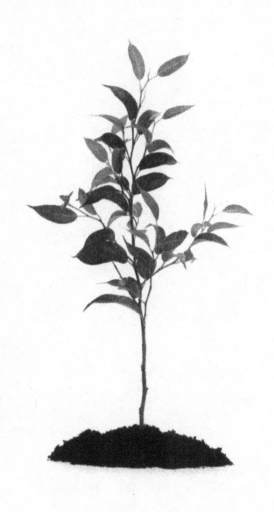

Chapter 5

Recovering *from* Traumatic Brain Injuries

Acceptance

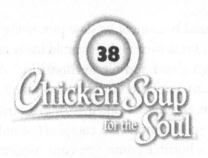

I Am Not My Brain Injury

If you must doubt something, doubt your limits.

~Price Pritchett

I n the fall of 2009, while making my way home from a conference, I was rear-ended on a major interstate. A brain injury was one of the many things I was left to deal with in the aftermath of my accident.

It might seem like an obvious statement, but there's nothing quite like your brain. Personally, I took mine for granted until I lost its full functionality. Since that time, I've learned that in good health my brain keeps everything running in good order. When the brain is broken, however, it operates more like a cruel time machine. After mine was injured, I found myself stuck in some memories, while unable to retain new ones for more than a few days. My emotions were scrambled and I would flip-flop back and forth between wanting to laugh and wanting to cry. More often than not, I felt like I'd been transported back to my childhood brain.

As you can imagine, an experience like this is quite frightening. Prior to my accident, I had performed at a high level. I had always been an outstanding student throughout school. I worked at a well-paying advertising executive position, enjoyed freelance writing and served in several leadership roles through my church and community. But now, it felt like all was lost. I had entered the twilight zone of life without a proper brain. I could barely speak a straight sentence. My brain seemed to move like an old computer that you have to wait for after every command because of its slow processing speed. The doctors told me I couldn't drive and that I would likely never work again. "You should just go ahead and file for disability," they encouraged. The list of "You Can't Do's" and "You'll Never's" went on and on.

Initially, it was easy to succumb to their disheartening prognoses for my life. I felt so abnormal and completely unlike myself. I felt like the victim of a horrible crime. Someone recklessly hit me and I would never be the same. I spiraled into a long grieving process, but when I came out on the other side of it, I was at ground zero. I had a fresh place to build from. In fact, there was nowhere for me to go in life other than forward.

The only way I could manage to restart was to take life in little bite-sized chunks. I was easily fatigued and overwhelmed, which if allowed to go too far, always resulted in a tear-filled meltdown. "Oh, Mom didn't get her nap today," I recall my kids saying when witnessing one of my weary, brain injury-induced tantrums. The only way I could manage was to take small steps. Like the old cliché says, "One step forward, two steps back," and this was true for me much of the time. I would begin easy workouts to regain my strength and balance, for example, only to discover that I had grossly irritated my neck injury, which I had also sustained in the accident. This would end in an excruciating migraine. It was a painful and frustrating cycle that often seemed pointless.

It would have been much easier to just give up and give in. Instead, as I succeeded in one area, I found the courage to hobble another inch forward. As the rubble was gradually cleared away, more light began to permeate the situation. Something inside me changed. It was as though I had an inner cheerleader, an advocate of some sort, rallying me to continue on. At times, it literally felt like death was encroaching upon me. Not that I was dying, but that little by little, surgeries, doctors' appointments, and words of doom and gloom were constantly trying to overshadow me.

It was at my darkest point that the voice inside me seemed to become the loudest. "Hey, you are not your brain injury," I swore I heard one day. It was like an epiphany that motivated me to new heights. "I am not my brain injury. I'm not!" I repeated to myself, as the full power of its meaning soaked in. I was still a person, with a heart, a soul and emotions. While they might have been long shots for someone in my condition, I had new dreams and goals, too.

I had been blaming the other driver in the accident for robbing me of my life and he had been held accountable for his actions. However, I was the one who had been allowing my brain injury to define me. I came to see that when tragedy strikes, whether it's a car accident, divorce or grief, there is a tendency for these things to take over our lives. The pain can be so debilitating that it's only natural for anyone to become absorbed in the situation for a time. But, if left unattended, these things will eventually stake their claim on our identity.

This revelation helped me to understand that I still needed validation and support about the reality of my health situation, but if I wanted to truly move on, I would have to change my perspective. I then decided to see myself as a survivor. I had to acknowledge that I had experienced something and been changed by it. But going forward, it would need to just be another slice of the pie of my life. My brain injury would be one ingredient in the recipe, not the whole pie itself.

My paradigm shift thrust me onward through many obstacles. It's taken several years of ratcheting up my goals, but I am back at work full-time now. I drive and write again. I'm also probably in the best physical shape of my life, due to my dedication to regaining my health. I try to live each day to the fullest, being cautious not to take things, like my brain, for granted.

~Stephanie Davenport

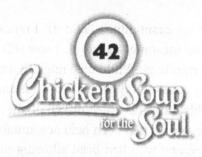

42

Right Where I'm Supposed to Be

Wherever the art of medicine is loved, there is also a love of humanity.

~Hippocrates

At about the five-year mark after my sixth concussion I received a request from my stepmother, Shirley, to answer a survey on Facebook. The questions on the survey were designed to help people get to know family and friends better, asking questions on topics not likely discussed in person. She and Dad had married in June of 2005, only two years before, so we were still getting to know each other.

The one survey question that really got my attention was, "If you could be anywhere in the world right now, where would you want to be?" My first inclination was to pick one of the locations on my bucket list. Then I gave the question a little more thought and realized there was only one right answer: I am right where I am supposed to be.

In February 2002 I was spending a long weekend at Winter Park, Colorado. The conditions were icy, so I had not skied all weekend. But with a few inches of fresh snow the morning of my scheduled departure, I ventured onto the slopes, hoping to eke out a few good runs. Midway down the mountain on my first run, I stopped to enjoy the beautiful snowy scenery. While standing crossways on the slope, I somehow lost my balance and fell backwards, hitting my helmeted head on the icy ground that was barely cushioned by the new snow. I had an immediate headache, and while trying a second run I developed nausea, so I decided to call it quits and head back home.

I had an uneventful ninety-mile drive, but the next days and weeks were anything but uneventful. I had suffered a concussion, the end result of which was residual cognitive problems and issues with my vision. I spent weeks going to rehabilitation, didn't drive for almost eleven months, and couldn't fly my pride and joy, a four-seat Cherokee airplane. I had a ten month supervised return-to-work trial that was unsuccessful, ending my eighteen-year career as a physician, the last three in charge of a medium-sized medical clinic in Colorado.

Losing my medical career, as well as the relationships I had with my patients, coworkers and many friends post-TBI was difficult to deal with. I was also dealing with the possibility of permanently losing my ability to fly, as I had not been able to pass the Federal Aviation Administration's medical examination since my injury.

While I was actively recovering from my traumatic brain injury, in 2005 my father sustained his own TBI. Dad fell while climbing down from the roof of his motor home, where he'd been repairing a leak. He fell headfirst onto the ground. Initially, it appeared he had only wrenched his neck, but over the next days and weeks we learned he'd fractured his neck and sustained a TBI. Even though I couldn't practice medicine, I was able to act as the medical liaison for my family, interpreting complex test results and medical forecasts, making Dad's recovery go a little more smoothly for my stepmom. Ironically, my TBI had allowed me to be available to help care for Dad during his hospitalization, affirming my belief that I am right where I am supposed to be.

As time has gone on, it is even more evident that I am on the right life path. As a physician with a traumatic brain injury, I've had many opportunities to educate medical professionals, the lay community, people with brain injuries and their supporters and caregivers about dealing with the consequences of this devastating injury. This has led to the publishing of a book based on my presentations, which has helped countless additional people navigate this journey. As a practicing family doctor, I always loved educating patients and the community on health-related issues, so providing brain injury education continues to fulfill that passion for me.

I believe without a doubt that my traumatic brain injury was a gift. It didn't seem so at first, but it resulted in me being "Right Where I'm Supposed to Be."

~Cheryle Sullivan, MD

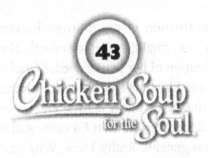

43

My Confession

A whole stack of memories never equal one little hope.
~Charles M. Schulz

My first confession about my disabilities was to my parents a few years after my car accident at age sixteen. Twenty years later, I'd tell my husband and children that my Jekyll and Hyde behavior had to do with my grief, my amnesia, my history, my deception and my lingering disabilities.

I didn't talk much about my head injury or my amnesia to anyone. Once I could fake my way through most situations, I was certain that I'd make it back to full recovery. So if my deception was caught in the missing details, I'd wave them off as if they no longer mattered. I'd remember one day... only I didn't.

I became experienced in the practice of sleight of hand and distraction. I wanted to stave off potential pity, close scrutiny and harsh judgment. I wanted people to like me for me. If not, I was happy being the odd girl out, or so I said. So when I came across my old box of journals, written during the worst of the amnesia, migraines, light sensitivity, etc., I made plans to destroy them. Surely my words were a crutch I no longer needed. They were a memento of the worst times of my life and their existence proved just how far I'd fallen. I should have gotten rid of them long ago.

No problem. I plotted to rid myself of the evidence of my hard luck. One rainy afternoon, I snuck upstairs and took care of my problem with a paper shredder.

Only the destruction of my journals backfired. My teen self reared up inside me, raging at her dismissal. No recognition? No fanfare? No celebration of her heroic deeds? Grief and regret spewed over my nice, quiet life. I alternately raged at others' good fortunes and wept at the unfairness of my failures and miseries.

It seemed I'd forgotten how far I'd come and what blessings surrounded me. I was grateful. Really, I was. Why couldn't I act like it?

A heart wants what it wants, and mine ached for goals never reached and dreams laid to rest prematurely. I marveled at my peers' accolades while I stayed at home by default. I didn't have the experience or education to catch up, so I was stuck. I understood the howling that burst forth from my soul. I'd hidden it for so long; it would not be silenced anymore.

I lived in the "It's not fair!" stage until I hated the feeling and how ungrateful it made me for all I'd accomplished. I won't say I don't ever visit that negative place—I do. When I find myself back there in the achingly slow, hard hours, I try to keep the visits short. Even in my deepest amnesia days, I knew the way forward wasn't back. Reclaiming isn't necessary for a good life; rebuilding is.

That's what my journals showed me. When you have nothing else, you have now. What are you going to do with it?

That's what my wise, brave teenaged self showed me in those journals. It's okay if you can't recall what you did last weekend or do what you did last year. What can you do now to make this day better?

My kids have become excellent storytellers. They recount our lives together for me so I can remember. I can't always hold onto those precious memories, but they can. It's good to share the good and bad with those you love.

I shudder to think what would have happened if I'd kept hiding my true nature from the people I care about most. And no matter what I can't do or be, I am here. In spite of everything, I am here.

So if I need to ask, "Can you tell me the story of your birthday party?" one more time, they will. That's what our loved ones do. They help us carry our burdens like they were precious cargo.

I have to remind myself I was hindered, but I overcame. Most importantly, I'm here now, and that's all that matters because here is where I most want to be. I've crafted a wonderful life in spite of setbacks. I have won.

~Donna Stamey Reeve

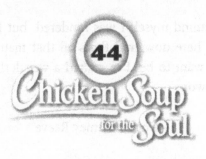

44

It's a Marathon Not a Sprint

I find hope in the darkest of days and focus in the brightest.
~Dalai Lama

"It's a marathon not a sprint." Whenever I heard those words, I always thought of world-class athletes running a grueling twenty-six-mile race. Today, those few words resonate quite differently with me. They were the first words told to me multiple times by my son's doctors and nurses when my son became a reluctant member of the traumatic brain injury club. Little did I know, my son and my family would be running the marathon of our lives.

During the early morning of May 27, 2012, twenty-three-year-old Richard was speeding, going over 100 miles an hour on the freeway. He over-corrected on a turn heading off the ramp. His car flipped three times. He was thrown forty feet from his car through the sunroof, landing in some bushes. He was not wearing a seatbelt.

Within seconds, my son, a national collegiate tennis player just beginning his studies at Arizona State University, was fighting for his life.

Luckily, the first responders arrived within minutes. Richard almost died three times in the ambulance but was revived. When he arrived at a level-one trauma center, the neurosurgeon performed an immediate craniotomy and took out a grapefruit-sized piece of bone from his skull to relieve the pressure from the swelling. His brain was bleeding from a hematoma, and he suffered a diffuse axonal injury, the shearing of parts of the brain. He also broke several vertebrae, shattered his hip, broke all of his ribs and suffered two collapsed lungs.

Doctors gave him little chance to survive the night, much less function cognitively because of the damage to the brain and spinal cord; the prognosis was that he would probably never walk again.

He survived the night, and this is where our marathon began. Myriad tubes and apparatuses surrounded my son so that I barely recognized him. My husband said I fell to my knees when the neurosurgeon said Richard would probably never walk again and would probably remain in a vegetative state. Our world was shattered within minutes.

Richard made it through the first few days and slowly opened his eyes, staring into space at something only he could see. Little by little, the life-sustaining tubes were extracted, and he breathed on his own with the help of a tracheotomy. Within three weeks, he underwent two brain surgeries and two spinal cord operations.

We were told in the beginning that all brain injuries are different and that patients do best with family support. The recovery process for brain injuries takes a very long time. Some doctors will give a two-year mark; however, research now shows that brain injury recovery can continue for years.

Our daily vigils with Richard began in the ICU while family and friends talked to him and played music. In time, he started mouthing the words to Blink 182's "Small Things" and James Blunt's "Beautiful." The nurses, angels in disguise, asked Richard to show them two fingers every day until finally two fingers were what he showed them. Although we were told that there were no nerve connections in his feet, we saw his toes move. Weeks later, he was moving his legs like a bucking bronco.

The marathon continued.

His next transition was to move to a specialty hospital to heal until he could enter an inpatient rehab unit. Here is where the trach came out, and we could hear his unique voice. He first started talking in numbers, but then, slowly, everyday conversations began. Brain-injured patients sometimes suffer from dysphasia where they mix up words. A cup may be called a table and a table may be called the number five.

The long days of Richard's recovery were some of my darkest. I did not know if my son would ever be the son I knew before. Would he have the same sense of humor? Would he walk again? Would he be able to get a job and live independently? Would he get married and have children of his own? I allowed myself to break down and cry. Then I scoured the Internet for success stories and got down on my knees and prayed.

Two months after his accident, Richard stood for the first time. Weeks later he took his first steps with the help of a walking apparatus. He had to laboriously learn to do everything all over again like a child — talking, walking, eating, brushing his teeth, showering, and walking to the bathroom. This took five months.

And the marathon continued.

Richard graduated to the inpatient rehab unit where his progress accelerated. It was not always easy to motivate him to get better, and at one time, we told him we would pay him ten dollars for each session of "stupid therapy" as he called it. Money was always a motivator for him. By the time he left the unit three months later, he could walk with a walker, get dressed by himself, and was working on his short-term memory. When the nurses asked where he was, he still did not know if he was in a hospital or a hotel. He had no idea what day it was or who the President was. Every day he begged to go home. He finally got his wish.

But the marathon wore on. At home he continued with his outpatient therapies and still used a feeding tube because his swallowing muscles were not strong enough to eat. At first I panicked about how I was going to work the feeding tube machine and was afraid I would starve him to death. We had our laughs when I would not quite get the feeding tube into the slot and the liquid would squirt all over him. But by December 2012, he could eat and drink again on his own. Slowly, his weight, which had plummeted to 140 pounds, climbed up to 200 pounds on his six-foot-five frame.

Since Richard needed complete twenty-four-hour supervision for a year, I became his best friend. We went everywhere together—the grocery store, doctors' visits, outpatient therapy, social security appointments, and the movies. It was a time period where he was re-learning social etiquette—brain-injured patients can be quite blunt. Luckily, his good friends stayed by his side to give me a reprieve. After all, does a twenty-something really want his mom to be his best friend?

After daily hard work, and with the help of his outpatient therapists, he can now run, play basketball, bowl, play tennis, read, write, and drive a car. In October 2013, his neuropsychological testing showed he still has deficits in short-term memory, processing information, and attention span. But he was told just a few days ago it is time for him to go back to college.

Over a year ago, I thought I had lost my son. I was clueless as to what recovery involved and hated that I was forced into the world of traumatic brain injury. But through a lot of education, help from amazing professionals, friends and family, a new normal emerged.

My tears are now not for me but for another mother who will watch her son or daughter begin his or her own marathon. Hope is the key. Our marathon still continues but it gets easier every day. I never liked sprints anyway.

~Sheri Siwek

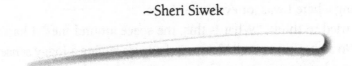

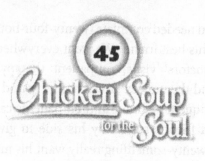

I Work!

The only journey is the one within.
~Rainer Maria Rilke

The white Ram Truck flew into the parking lot and screeched to a stop. A man jumped out and began screaming at me. His face was red with a rage I couldn't comprehend. I was standing next to my green Voyager holding a book. I couldn't see what he was carrying. He surged at me, his well-muscled arms swinging. He got right up in my face. I don't remember what happened after that.

I quit working.

Not only as in, I stopped going to my job. But as in I, the me that was me, just stopped functioning. I woke the next morning not knowing where I was, or even who I was.

I tried to think, "What is this, the space around me?" I had no idea. No associations at all. Scariest of all was having a foggy sense of my own identity, my sense of being a person. I touched my arms, my stomach. My head hurt. But who was I?

My husband was standing over the bed. "Good morning, Jan." Who was he? Why was he here? The voice sounded familiar. His face looked like one I had known but I couldn't put his face together with his name, Dave, much less with who he was: my husband.

Later, I was administered a mental status exam. I didn't know who the President was or what day it was. Not only could I not count backward from one hundred, I couldn't comprehend what a number was. It would take months and months for the abstract concept of numbers to make the least bit of sense to me.

Later, my two daughters came in. I didn't know who they were.

It was my second concussion in two months. The damage was done.

In the hours and days that followed, I still wasn't working. I didn't recognize faces, voices, places, or words written on a page. I couldn't comprehend what people said to me. I cried a lot. Out of frustration, anger, sadness, I stayed in bed and slept and cried. I couldn't focus on TV. I couldn't interact with my daughters because I didn't know what they were saying. Words were meaningless gibberish. I tried to read, but the sentences were blurs of indistinguishable marks on a page. Sound and light were intolerable. I lived alone in a darkened, silent cocoon.

Dave took me back to the doctor. I have no idea what she said.

Christmas came and we traveled from our home in Colorado to Minnesota to be with Dave's family. We drove all night and at dawn the girls made up a song, "Sunrise at St. Olaf." We all laughed. Then I retreated into my zone. I sat in a comfy chair in the corner of his parents' house in a haze, watching the festivities. I wasn't really there. I nodded and ate the traditional Swedish Christmas Eve smorgasbord and saw my girls open their gifts. They had gift cards to be used at the Mall of America. We went on the Kite-Eating-Tree ride. I remember how unreal it all felt.

As the months passed, I began to put some pieces together. Not remembering what had happened, I heard about it from an eyewitness. I cried. My job was gone.

Gradually, I began to resemble, at times, a normal person. I could almost fake it for brief periods.

I listened to quiet classical music. I asked for some simple books. I reconnected with the girls and found that making fun of my inability to do anything logical made for good humor. We played dominoes and laughed at my failure to count up my points at the end of the round. I ventured out with Dave to our daughter Kaia's basketball games. We went to our younger daughter Annika's choir concert. He had to guide me, hold my elbow, help me with steps, and navigate our way through the crowds. On my own, I froze.

I had always been a high achiever. I had the practical equivalent of a doctoral degree, hours of education in complex topics beyond my four-year master's. I had even directed a doctoral program. Highly accomplished and respected in my field, I could no longer function. I had written a book. Now I couldn't even read it.

As I became more aware of my situation and my disabilities I was humiliated. I hid out, taking solace only in my family.

And I began to take apart socks. Dave bought me packages of white socks and I methodically unraveled them. Stitch by stitch. Strand by strand until I had a mound of white thread beside my bed that came up to the level of the mattress. The girls worried about this phase. It was an obsession. I'd never been obsessive before but had always doodled. I found I couldn't do that anymore but I could unravel socks. The thread mounded up and around the bed until even I had to agree it was ridiculous. Eventually, I found pillow covers at a craft bazaar and stuffed them with the unraveled socks.

Dave was both father and mother to the girls for a time. He took over the cooking because not only could I not multitask, I couldn't even task. I couldn't do processes that required thinking in steps. I could chop onions but I couldn't manage the many pieces required to put a complete meal on the table.

More than anything, I was angry. I was angry at the man who hurt me, the events that led up to the attack. And I was angry at God. Faith had always been an essential part of my life. I got through a challenging childhood by remembering the promise I'd heard as a young girl: "I have come that you might have life and have it abundantly." (Jesus, from John 10:10) What happened to that abundant life? It was stolen from me, I felt, and I was furious. My time to enjoy the precious moments of daily life with my daughters was stolen. My delightful relationship with Dave was stolen. It had all become a chore, something to get through. I was haunted by nightmares. I was haunted by fear that my attacker would return. I was angry at God for letting all this happen.

Time passed. My brain was healing from the inside out. I began to feel more and more like myself. I found a good therapist who helped me process the trauma. I looked at life and wanted back in.

I read about what attacks like the one I experienced do to people. I gained some perspective on the dynamics of my injury. I stopped unraveling socks.

The best thing is that I started trusting again. Trusting (most) people. Trusting myself. I was so ashamed that I had "let" this happen to me; I came to see it was not my fault. And not God's either.

We celebrated Easter. New life. New possibilities. From the strands of life left over from the injury, I found a new vocation: being a friend. Simple. No advanced degree required. People need good, faithful friends. I can do that. I work!

~Anneli Norrland

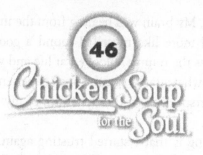

46

Building a Tree House

All things must come to the soul from its roots, where it is planted.
~Saint Teresa of Avila

Labor Day, the last hurrah of summer. The kids were in the tree looking for the perfect branches on which to build a tree house. They were so young, and no one ever thought to tell the children not to reach out toward a power line. But my adventurous daughter Christina did just that and 4800 volts of electricity catapulted her thirty feet to the ground. She lost consciousness as her clothes and flesh began to burn. I was worried that she might not survive the fall and the burns. I never thought about a possible traumatic brain injury.

Christina was angry because the first responders wanted her to have an IV; it took four men to hold her down. Once at the ER, I heard the word "electrocution" for the first time. I hadn't quite processed what had actually happened to her. Meanwhile, I had to make sure that my older daughter Rebecca was told by an adult what had happened and have someone care for her. I was overwhelmed, but I had no idea how much my life had changed in that split second.

At the hospital, I could hear Christina scream as she was put into a shower to clean the dirt, grass and leaves off her body. The nurses needed to give her morphine during the shower to better handle the pain. I still hadn't cried.

Christina would have a total of three surgeries, each on a Wednesday. The first was to thoroughly clean her wounds, the second was for skin grafts and the third was to take out all the staples. Her nurse said that as the surgeon walked into the OR, Christina broke out in song with the "Hallelujah Chorus"—what a kid!

Christina eventually made it back to school. Rebecca seemed to be doing well also, but was at a loss how to deal with Christina and all the medical attention she needed. Life seemed to slip into a routine, but centered on medical and therapy appointments, as well as special baths for Christina. Rebecca felt ignored by everyone around her.

Christina seemed to be adjusting to school. She received extra help with language as well as physical concerns. But I was noticing she was less even-tempered than she was previously. I thought perhaps it was part of the normal recovery from the accident. But then puberty struck. Christina became unmanageable. She would run away, fight with others at school, and refuse to do her work. Even though she had a one-on-one aide at the middle school, she would hit others (including me.) She even threatened suicide.

Seemingly overnight, she had become a person I did not know. Our lives were upside down again. Christina spent many days in mental health facilities. She was diagnosed with bipolar disorder, and although I kept saying she has a traumatic brain injury, no one wanted to listen to me. The police were at our house nearly every week and would end up transporting Christina to either a detention center or a mental health hospital.

Eventually, Christina went to live with her father in a nearby city. This did not help either. It seemed her father had less control than I did, and now teen shelters were added to her places of residence. Eventually, she came back to my home and was assigned a county social worker. In fact the county at one point took guardianship of her and placed her in another residential treatment center, this time long term. Christina flourished with 24/7 care and structure. She began school again and was doing well. However, because she was doing so well, she was released home. Her behavior escalated again. She ran away for days at a time and engaged in a number of illegal, inappropriate behaviors.

The calm, new normal we had developed as a family had unraveled. We kept all the knives in the house locked in the trunk of the car. I had to hire local college students to sit with Christina at night while I was at work if Rebecca was gone. Rebecca was getting ready to graduate from high school and enroll in college; she was being ignored again. Rebecca was embarrassed by her sister's behaviors. I didn't blame her. I was embarrassed, too. I felt guilty because I didn't know what to do to help the situation.

Before the accident, Christina was very social, very talkative and had a lot of friends. After the accident, her impulsiveness and erratic behaviors affected her ability to establish and keep friendships, and to get along with others.

Having a traumatic brain injury can be difficult. Generally, someone with a TBI does not look any different than anyone else. However, once you talk with her, you might notice something a little off. This made it harder to get support services for Christina—she looks like a typical twenty-year-old, with long blond hair, a winning smile and an engaging personality.

Our lives changed when Christina was electrocuted. It took me about a month to reach out to friends for support. I was so overwhelmed with the daily routine of being a single mom and trying to be there for both the girls that I did not take time for myself. I eventually did reach out to friends, family and my church. I would sit in the quiet pews and cry, but also feel hope: hope that everything would get better.

And it has. With time and persistence and the love of family, Christina is now growing into the young adult she can be. She is beginning to believe in herself again. She is the nurturing, caring individual whom everyone loves. Now she can talk about the accident without too much regret about what she used to be able to do and no longer can.

This life-changing experience provided a foundation from which to grow, to develop understanding, to begin seeing people for who they are. I want to believe that I am more open-minded, that I look beyond the initial first impression. I ask people how they are doing and really listen. I am more empathetic when talking with parents about concerns they may be having in their families. I have found that everyone has concerns; a personal or family difficulty that is hidden from others yet is a burden for them. Being available to listen, to offer a helping hand, can go a long way for that individual and also give purpose and meaning to our lives.

The tree house was never built. The tree was eventually cut down. However, the roots of caring for others, the roots of our family, are strong.

~Jan Heinitz

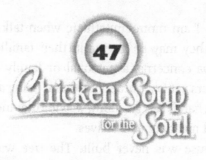

47

The Broken Hat

Never lose an opportunity of seeing anything beautiful,
for beauty is God's handwriting.
~Ralph Waldo Emerson

The first chill came early this year, and I was less than prepared for it. Waking up to an unexpectedly frosty morning, I frantically sorted through the tote of winter accessories to locate my son's furry trapper hat and mittens to ensure his warmth for the trip down the driveway to meet his school bus. As I was securing the chinstrap of his hat, Ryan pulled the big furry bill over his eyes. I well remember many tugs on that bill last winter, as he attempted to remove the hat but instead caused the threads securing the bill to his forehead to break and unravel. I internally scolded myself for not mending his broken hat before packing it away for the season. There wasn't enough time to do anything about it before school, so I sent him on his way with the furry bill hovering over his eyes and blocking his vision.

While running errands that day, I found an excellent deal on another trapper hat at a local consignment store. I smiled, believing I was being a good mom by resolving the broken hat problem. The next morning I dressed Ryan in his new hat. It fit perfectly, but I noticed that he was a bit fussy, and he attempted to remove it using his old "pull the bill" technique. I wrote off this unhappiness as his typical response to having anything on his head. The hat was secure, he was warm, and I could see his beautiful eyes gazing at me as I wheeled him down the driveway to meet the bus.

The day passed and I didn't give another thought to the new hat until I met him at the foot of the driveway at the end of his school day. As we were getting him onto the wheelchair lift, Mary, the bus attendant, mentioned that Ryan had been very somber on the trips to and from school. She jokingly suggested that we switch back to the old hat. After I brought Ryan inside, unbundled him, and removed him from his wheelchair, I read the daily notes from school and discovered that he had experienced a rare bad day. His teacher indicated that he had been sad all day instead of his normal animated self. I started to wonder if his mood was actually linked to the hat.

The next morning I dressed him in his old broken hat. He immediately started playing with the bill and pulling it over his eyes. His primary motivation for wearing his hat was to play, and he had adapted his old hat to suit his purpose. When Ryan saw Mary, he immediately initiated his peek-a-boo ritual with her. He was all smiles and laughter as we loaded him onto the bus. As expected, he had a great day at school, completely enjoying his interactions with his teachers, aides, and peers. He came home dancing for joy in his wheelchair. It turns out that the hat wasn't broken after all. It was exactly as it was meant to be, providing the optimal combination of warmth and play.

Life with Ryan has been full of many learning moments, and the hat story is but one of them. It is, however, the perfect metaphor for my son. Ryan's life forever changed close to twelve years ago. Born a typical baby, he was violently shaken at nine months of age by his daycare provider and suffered a massive traumatic brain injury. His expansive medical chart documents a life of physical brokenness. Ryan has severe quadriplegia and is unable to sit, stand, crawl, or walk without intervention and support. His high tone and spasticity have severely compromised his muscle and bone growth. He has a seizure disorder and frequently experiences a variety of other neurological quirks. He has cortical vision impairment, is hypersensitive to sound, and is orally fixated. All of his food must be puréed to avoid choking, and liquids must be thickened to prevent aspiration. Cognitively, he has profound learning challenges and he is non-verbal. Ryan is not able to perform any activities of daily living without assistance. While there are aspects of his brain and body that are fully intact, there are numerous complex gaps that make understanding his potential a challenge to physicians, therapists, educators, and virtually anyone who interacts with him, even, at times, us.

His injury initially caused an emotional breakdown in our family as we dealt with the anger, grief, and loss of trust associated with being victims of a violent crime. As we were dealing with the medical questions surrounding Ryan's life-threatening injury, we were also thrown into the midst of a criminal investigation, one in which our family interactions were scrutinized beyond measure and we were treated with rudeness and suspicion until ruled out as perpetrators of the crime. The road to healing and forgiveness was a long and difficult one, but through it all, Ryan set the tone for how our family should live. He chose to embrace life and finds delight in all of its blessings. We have followed his lead.

Ryan came close to dying from his brain injury. I fully believe that the child who eventually woke from coma was reborn. There was no road map for recovery, as brain injury is characterized by its mystery and unpredictability. His slate was wiped clean, and he was given the opportunity to completely define himself. All typical milestones were no longer applicable. There are things that Ryan will never be able to do, but by the grace of God he does not miss what he does not have. I know that he feels complete in who he is. As his personality has developed through the years, I have been frequently undone by the beauty that I have witnessed in him. He is so loving, joyful, and pure. If angels are among us, he is most definitely one. I have no doubt that God's purpose for him is profound. Ryan has drawn people together and inspired sensitivity, understanding, kindness, and generosity. His story is an ongoing voice for awareness of child abuse. He is evidence that despite significant obstacles one can achieve the seemingly unreachable through patience and hard work. He daily spreads abundant happiness and affection to all who interact with him, and his radiant smile is completely contagious. These are just a few of his accomplishments, but they are in my opinion milestones that many of us will never achieve. He is a hero and an ongoing miracle in our midst, and I am incredibly blessed to be his mom.

Through Ryan, I have learned that brokenness is a matter of perception. It is the amazing individual who can rise above his limitations and create a reality of completeness from that which would leave most of us permanently defeated. I am not saying that life with brain injury is easy. It is not, but we are passionate and deliberate in how we live it out. My son is anything but broken. He is as unique, beautiful, and as perfect as his hat.

~Kirsten Corrigan

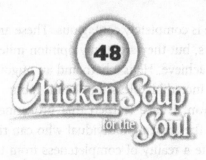

48

Finding the Glorious

The ultimate measure of a person is not where they stand in moments of comfort and convenience, but where they stand in times of challenge and controversy.

~Martin Luther King, Jr.

It has been six and a half years since I had a life-changing head injury from a car accident. It felt like being catapulted into a vast sense of nowhere, inner connections shattered. I have been rebuilding ever since. I had to learn how to move, think, feel, behave, and even interpret gravity all over again.

It's funny and serious at the same time. When you have a brain injury, what you use to interpret the world is not working properly, so you are not able to have an accurate sense of how injured you are. You have no idea—literally, because you don't have the neural connections *to* have that idea. You don't know that there is an issue until it shouts hello from the rooftops of your life through ongoing significant challenges for you and often everyone around you, too. I understand why caregivers I've spoken with have said, "It's like the person disappears." It is true. You may be there physically, yet the whole you that used to be there can't show up in this world because you don't have the wiring to do so, until hopefully, the connections are rebuilt.

When your ability to function collapses around you, you lose your sense of yourself. It is then, amidst the rubble, that you have the opportunity to build a new way of being by choice. It will look and feel different. But, different can be better. What if they couldn't put Humpty Dumpty back together again because they were trying to put him back together like he was, not like he was now designed to be?

What does it feel like for some of us with traumatic brain injury? If you can, imagine having a box in front of you that is about a foot wide and you want to pick it up. However, your hands stay three feet apart, so there are one-foot gaps between your hands and the box. If your brain is well enough, you can tell there are gaps. If it's not, you might only be able to see that the box is not moving, if you can even comprehend that. I found that it was only from asking others around me for supportive feedback that I began to understand what my "slides on a banana peel" looked like and then use that information to change my life via therapists and my own actions.

The accident happened on May 9, 2007, at 7:30 a.m. I was driving in fast-moving rush hour traffic. The skies were a cloudless blue and the roads beneath me were dry. Then everyone came to a stop except for the driver behind me. Slam! I learned what it means when "life changes in an instant." A big commercial truck rear-ended my vehicle at an estimated forty to fifty miles per hour.

I had to learn in great part to talk, read and write again. It was two years before I could read a book. I love Maya Angelou's writing and was drawn to her book *Letter to My Daughter*. When I opened it I found that it had short chapters, wide spacing and non-serif font so I gave it a try and it worked! To simplify the visual input even further, I would cover the opposite page and part of the page I was reading with a clean white sheet to compensate for my reduced level of cognitive processing. A friend of mine told me that before the accident I talked so fast she couldn't keep up with me; after the accident I spoke so slowly she couldn't remember what I'd last said.

One of the greatest challenges has been and still is my extreme sensory sensitivity. In the beginning I could not process any amount of visual input: sound, movement, or vibration. The only place that my nervous system would begin to relax was in a completely dark and silent room, a controlled environment hard to come by in this noisy, bustling world. The sounds of the heat coming on in the house, the flushing of a toilet, were nerve-wracking. Water running from the faucet into the metal kitchen sink was like thunder pounding in my head. I would shut the water off and lie down on the floor in tremors allowing my body and brain to reintegrate enough for the tremors to subside. I would rest there on the kitchen floor until I felt well enough to make my way to my bed, crawl into the haven of my sheets and pray for more recovery.

It was three months before I realized I didn't have my sense of humor. The fact that I could realize this was a huge step forward. Upon recognizing this I intently told the "construction crew" of my brain to get to work! I visualized connections being rebuilt and spent time feeling and watching this happening. It took about six months before my sense of humor started to come back. Humor is a great tool for making it through life, especially challenging times. I have spent years now with ear filters, noise-cancelling headphones, and dark sunglasses as needed to compensate for my sensory sensitivity.

Some of what has made it possible for me to continue to move forward today includes the grace of time and space coupled with large doses of love, patience, forgiveness, fortitude, releasing the challenges, grieving as needed, and a continual openness to see and receive the light at the end of many tunnels.

My cognitive therapist shared with me that most of her clients over time have said that their brain injury was one of the greatest gifts they had ever received. I am starting to see this as I continue my recovery: the gifts of being able to listen to music, to dance, to sing, to spend time with friends, to exercise, to appreciate life. What incredible, amazing, outrageously magnificent selves we are to live, breathe and function as human beings. We have no idea how absolutely stunningly capable we are and how glorious and scrumptious this world is when we connect with it inside and out.

~Kim Conrad

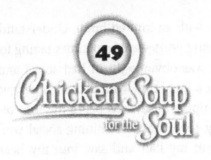

49

To Soar

Refuse to be average. Let your heart soar as high as it will.
~Aiden Wilson Tozer

It was just eleven days past my nineteenth birthday. I was in labor and all was not well. With forceps assist, Justin was finally delivered. Four weeks later, we were back at the hospital in the emergency room. The consequences of my ignorance in 1971, and a doctor's misdiagnosis, resulted in a vast array of consequences that have lasted to this day.

The traumatic delivery caused a slow leak in Justin's brain, a subdural hematoma. It did not show up for a couple of weeks. I recognized something was not quite right, but a doctor said I was overreacting and that Justin was just coming down with a cold. A week later, I could not wake him up and rushed him to the emergency room.

Most of the doctors trying to help my baby survive seemed harsh and abrupt toward me. I soon understood why. Justin's father and I were interrogated as to whether or not we had been violent with him. They kept asking if we had shaken Justin, or if we had accidentally dropped him.

It was the early 1970's. Justin's father and I were gentle peace freaks. We wanted to make a better world. We wanted to be great parents. Hurting our baby was incomprehensible to us.

The doctors initially reported that Justin had a 1 in 2,000 chance of surviving, let alone being anywhere near normal. Justin did survive, and thrived even with an injured brain. Understandably, all was not perfect. Justin's early years were sometimes taxing for us.

Early on, it was obvious Justin had social and developmental problems. I spent a lot of time with doctors, many who looked at my non-conformist hippie lifestyle as being the root of some of Justin's woes. Thankfully, there was one shining social worker who looked past the flowers in my hair and saw into my heart. She probably saved my sanity. Having one compassionate person offer loving kindness was worth fifty disdainful others who did not take the time to know me.

At three years of age, Justin was diagnosed as borderline autistic. He was hyperactive and not always responsive to interactions with other people. His speech skills were slow to develop. He had mild cerebral palsy. The compassionate social worker helped me map out some helpful developmental strategies, one of which included having Justin spend time with other children. I got a part-time job and put Justin in the best daycare I could find. Eventually, because of his tendency to throw things and clobber the other kids, he was asked to leave the program.

I spent a lot of time reading to Justin, trying to help him focus. He had to be under observation all the time, as he lacked survival skills. He would not just wander off, he would run. To relax us both, I would drive him to a construction site, or to the local airport, where he would sit in the car and watch the big machines that fascinated him. I used that time to read novels. As Justin's motor skills improved, he focused on mechanical toys. His favorite toy was a riding, pedal tractor. He was at his best in quiet surroundings, in motion.

Over the years, I searched for help and guidance wherever I could find it. My exterior became less radical, and I was not so frequently accused of being the cause of his problems. After a few years, I decided to earn a college degree to help save the environment. The local university had a daycare center, so I enrolled Justin. They were wonderful folks and helped to find solutions to problems rather than pointing fingers. The head professor even visited my home to observe Justin. He was totally amazed at the compliant, focused, gentle boy who was so much different than the one he saw at the daycare center.

When Justin started elementary school, the teachers worked with me the best they could. This was the era when the education system was just beginning to give specialized help to children with special needs. One astute teacher observed that Justin sometimes intentionally committed infractions so that he would be put in the time-out room. It seemed that the more people and activity around him, the more stressed he felt. He had difficulty processing classroom instructions, distracted by a group. One on one, he thrived.

I also searched for activities that would engage and center Justin's attention. Computers intrigued him. By eight, he was learning to write simple programs on his VIC-20 computer. Justin always loved flying machines. He had an innate understanding of aerodynamics. We had long conversations where he would explain the function of things like canards. He wanted to be a pilot. His colorblindness, cerebral palsy, and the seizures that started when he was twelve, precluded that aspiration... sort of.

As a young man, Justin earned two computer-related associate's degrees. While in school, he worked part-time as a bagger at a grocery store. It was routine work that involved predictable interactions with people. After college, unable to find a job in the computer field, he continued to bag groceries. He lived spartanly and saved his money.

Justin became friends with a compassionate man who saw past his idiosyncrasies and shared his passion for flying. They started flying remote-controlled planes together.

Today, as a middle-aged man, Justin still bags groceries for a living. It is a routine job with low stress and great predictability. It is comfortable. He earns enough money to live in a nice apartment, and manages his finances well enough to fund his hobbies.

One of his hobbies is to build small robots from scratch and program them to do simple tasks. But his main passion remains flying. He worked hard and earned a rating to fly a paraglider. Most people would find it extremely stressful to hang in the air on just the wind. But to Justin, it is simple freedom. He now soars in the thermals where he can fly free, above all other external over-stimulation. And that is how I like to think of my son: soaring!

~Jane Marie Allen Farmer

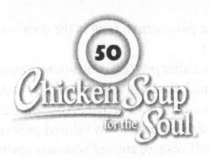

50

The Dance

Dancing with the feet is one thing, but dancing with the heart is another.
~Author Unknown

Yellow light from the windows of the ballroom on the second floor of the Lenox Community Center pierced the cold darkness. I hurried down the street toward the sounds of the music from the contra dance band playing inside. I felt a sense of anticipation and joy for the dance and then the familiar, sinking question gnawed at my heart—would I be able to do it?

Contra dancing had long been my passion. It is a type of New England folk dance set to lively Anglo-Celtic music played by a live band. It provides a positive social environment, wonderful exercise, and an evening's entertainment all rolled up in one. The dance is arranged in long lines of paired couples, each progressing to dance with another couple as the figure is completed. By the time each specific dance is over, one will have danced with many smiling people. At the end, you thank your current partner and find another partner for the next dance! A "caller" announces the moves. The caller teaches the dance and then gives cues during the first segments of the particular dance. But soon folks realize they are dancing without the caller's voice, responding as one to the joyful beat of the music. For me, a night of contra dance was a perfect evening.

Until I sustained a traumatic brain injury, that is. My life changed in an instant, the instant that my head came in contact with a metal doorjamb. It was simple enough: I was going to a meeting with colleagues and the pavement in front of the door was uneven. Life as I knew it was over.

For a few years after my TBI, contra dancing was not even in my awareness. It seemed that I had forgotten the joy of dance. I was more focused on relearning the basic activities of daily living. At first, I was simply determined to get back to my beloved profession of nursing. I had no ability to self-observe and see what was obvious to the people who really knew me. I was a different person. I was lucky enough to look the same and could fool most people who didn't really know me. In fact, I could even fool myself. It took several years to get to the point of beginning to understand what happened to my brain on that November day.

About two years after my TBI, I found myself back at the contra dance. I sat and watched the dancers. The music was too loud and the movement made me dizzy. There was too much going on there, too much stimulation. My brain was not able to process all that was happening around me. Unable to tolerate it, I sadly went home. Many months later, I went again, and this time I tried to dance. For a gal who was used to dancing every dance, one dance was enough, but it was a start. I was beginning to find my dancing feet again.

The more I learned about the journey of recovery from TBI, the better able I was to come up with some strategies. A rested brain is essential. I had to take a nap before going to the dance. It was not necessary to dance every dance; pacing was important. Keeping well hydrated was also critical. Taking a break from the stimulation by going outside into the quiet darkness and letting my brain "reboot" was helpful. Most importantly, recognizing when I was "finished" and going home was not a failure, it was another success in embracing my "new normal."

That Saturday evening, I decided to take a break and sat out a dance. I watched the dancers in the lines before me, and found my attention drawn to a slender woman with short salt and pepper hair. She had a different way of dancing. Her moves were very angular and brisk and her face showed great concentration on what she was doing. What she lacked in agility and grace, she made up for in determination and spirit. If she stumbled, she got back into the line and kept dancing. It was obvious to me that she was an experienced dancer, despite her challenges.

I found my way to her at the intermission and introduced myself. "I am so moved by your love of dance and your courage," I said. She introduced herself as Jenn. We spoke for a few minutes. Then, I listened with fascination as she shared her own TBI story.

"When I was a high school senior, I suffered a traumatic brain injury. My first memory after my accident was waking up two months later in a hospital bed in Woburn, Massachusetts. I was apparently in a rehabilitation hospital teaching my body how to live again.

"I loved to contra dance, but at that point, I could hardly stand, let alone dance. After about four months, my dad took me to a monthly contra dance to watch. I sat on the stage with the band and followed the dancers with my eyes. After a year, I was sort of waltzing again. After about two years, I went to a small contra dance in Fitzwilliam, New Hampshire. I knew everyone there: the caller, the musicians and most of the dancers. Toward the end of the evening, the caller called 'Money Musk.' The musicians played the tune slowly, and the dancers helped me dance my first contra dance since the accident. That moment filled me with such joy and sense of accomplishment that from then on you couldn't stop my dancing!

"My dancing ability now depends on many factors: how tired I am, how fast the music is, what the dance is, and who is in the contra line. The dancers who know me know how to dance with me, but a lot of the new dancers aren't quite sure what to do when they reach me in line. I, however, just kind of bull my way through and eventually I'll reach someone who knows me and I can 'regroup' and dance on!"

• • •

That night, I found a new teacher, a new guide in my recovery from TBI. I learned how important it is to rediscover those things, like music and dance, which are truly meaningful in life, those things that feed the soul. I learned that I needed to trust those around me: professionals, family and friends alike, my "dancers in the line" to provide the structure and feedback needed to refine the new me. I learned the importance of finding strategies to allow for my challenges and provide the possibility of success in trying different activities after TBI. I learned that taking a well-considered leap of faith is important, that I do not want to have fear of failure define me on this journey. I learned that life is seldom all or nothing... that I do not have to dance every dance... that joy is not dependent upon perfection. And I learned that I can indeed do it, not perhaps in the way that I had done it before, but I can do it!

On a cold Saturday night, in a little New England town, two women met by chance at a contra dance. They shared their experience, courage and hope, by both words and example. On this journey of recovery from traumatic brain injury, it is a wonderful thing to "dance like no one is watching." In fact, it is true of life in general. Dare to find your joy... and keep dancing, no matter what your dance might be!

~Helen Reid Stewart

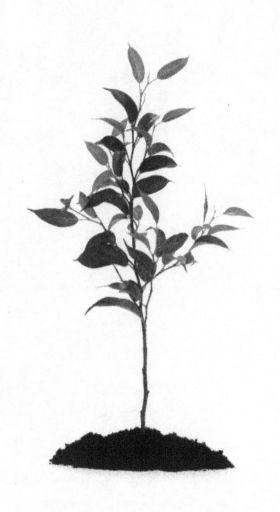

Chapter 6

Recovering *from* Traumatic Brain Injuries

A Family Affair

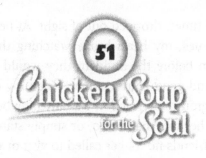

It's Personal

A single rose can be my garden... a single friend my world.
~Leo Buscaglia

Day after day, I asked myself the same question. Are people callous toward those with disabilities or do they just feel helpless? It has taken me a long time to realize that most feel powerless and uncomfortable. Even so, when one by one all of my adult daughter's friends disappeared, it didn't ease the hurt and disappointment.

It has been eighteen months since my daughter suffered a traumatic brain injury after falling down the basement stairs. She was given little chance to survive. But, through surgery, and later, therapy at a rehab hospital, she miraculously lived and is physically fit and as beautiful as ever. She was blessed in this regard and we choose to focus on this instead of dwelling on the significant cognitive problems and not just a speech impairment with which she still struggles.

I've learned to deal with the speech and cognitive issues myself, but the reaction from her friends has been tough. I admit it is difficult to have a conversation with her, as she doesn't always understand what people are saying and tries to sort it out by asking them questions again and again. It takes patience, I know.

At first, she was surrounded by friends who offered encouragement and support. But once they met her for lunch or talked to her at their children's school events, they began to vanish. One of her friends called and arranged to take her to work out at the gym, but after a couple of times, dropped out of sight. At her son's basketball and baseball games, my heart broke watching the other mothers ignore her, when before the accident they would sit with her and enjoy laughter and good conversation. When my daughter tried to be a part of the group, the reaction was anything but compassionate. They would tell her they had to go, or simply stare at her. It wasn't long before her friends no longer called to visit or go places. Within a few months, she was left without friends and even lost primary custody of her son when his father cited her deficiencies in court.

For me, it has taken months, and I admit it is still a constant struggle to give her friends the benefit of the doubt. After all, when she walks into a room, no one would ever suspect there is anything wrong with her—that is, until she talks. Maybe they were afraid they'd say something wrong. Or it could be that they didn't want to be bothered. My emotions bounced from one explanation to the other, wishing I'd been prepared for this. But human nature can never be predicted.

I suffered from a combination of hurt, bitterness and the emotions of a lioness trying to protect her cub. I wanted to strangle them and scream, "Have you no compassion? How would you want to be treated if you were in this position? Can't you see she needs you now more than ever?" I was indignant. As far as I was concerned, this was prejudice towards the disabled.

Days and weeks stretched into months with no word from her friends. Then, one day, a friend from childhood whom she hadn't seen for many years began calling. My heart swelled with gratitude. She came by weekly and took my daughter for walks, shopping, and lunch. I marveled at the gesture, and it was heartwarming to see my daughter's eyes light up each week. The woman treated her the same as she always had, as if nothing were amiss. She didn't talk over her but straight to her, and seemed unfazed by any deficits.

Today, my daughter is making a new life for herself, surrounded by a supportive family and a few new friends plus her loyal childhood friend. She volunteers, works out at the local gym, and participates in her son's school activities—even though many people are reserved around her.

For me, I've learned that you can't make people do what you want them to. But most of all I've learned to take things one day at a time and to focus on the positive, like that dear friend who chose to help instead of withdrawing. Even though I have tried to tell her, she will never truly know what a difference she has made just being there for us, reminding us that there are folks out there who overlook deficiencies and focus on friendship.

~Arlene Rains Graber

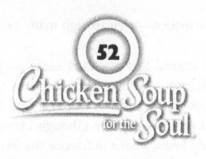

Making Believe

I think we may safely trust a good deal more than we do.
~Henry David Thoreau

It was late October when my husband Miles, a tree crew lead, was hit in the forehead by an eighty-pound branch when a tree fell the wrong way. After surgery and in-patient rehab, he was released, and though they called his traumatic brain injury mild, he came home a shell of the man I knew, a shadow of the daddy our two young children trusted.

The holiday season arrived and I forged ahead optimistically, fueled by the adrenaline of survival. Relatives sent a package full of gift cards from what seemed like a thousand different retailers. Friends came by with dinner. The children, three and five, gave everyone hope in their cute pictures with Santa. Meanwhile my husband, who couldn't remember names, missed conversational nuances and slept the day away.

In the hospital, I saw the scan showing which part of the brain had bled, the left frontal lobe a dusty nebula. "The frontal lobe controls your executive functioning," a nurse practitioner told me. I could scarcely eke out a question, not wanting to know the answer. She explained how executive function helps us connect past experience with present action. Her list sounded like prerequisites for normal living: planning, memory, attention, problem solving, verbal reasoning, and mental flexibility. My sleepy inner contrarian woke up. Did she mean to predict his future? Wasn't the brain mostly untapped, its plasticity an open book? I dug in my heels, refusing to believe Miles's cognition would be limited.

Six years later, I recognize these as the arguments of trauma. I thought that because we were living idyllic lives, with beautiful children, a nice house, and good jobs, that we could beat the odds. My attitude was: persist and conquer. Perseverance did help, and Miles improved. And yet during the darkest days, when he struggled with a seizure disorder and growing despondency over joblessness, I learned how lying is sometimes a necessary defense.

Trauma compartmentalizes life into before and after. Before the accident, people at work knew me as a friendly front desk girl. Immediately after, I was a brave wife and mother, quickly promoted to full-time staff. My colleagues wanted the inside scoop on Miles's impressive survival, so I spoon-fed them my meal of malarkey, explaining how he had vision problems, and we weren't sure what he'd be doing for work, but that one thing was for sure: he'd dodged a bullet. My defensive armor was so intact that I take the blame for what happened next, during a routine Monday morning staff meeting. On my way to the conference room, the Chief Financial Officer pulled me aside and said, "I'd like to give you a few minutes to address the staff." I was stunned. Was I supposed to talk about my department's latest project? "No, no," she told me. "We want to hear about Miles."

You do not say no to a genuine request from a person of power. Come my turn, my hands were a shaking mess. I took the microphone and gushed about how my colleagues had been so generous to take up the slack in my absence. I thanked everyone for contributing to the home meal-delivery service. Then came the biggest fib of my life. "Miles is..." Deep breath. "...about ninety percent toward making a full recovery." I hadn't planned on it, but there it was, a bold-faced lie, and a cacophony of clapping followed as my reward. Whereas I should have stomped and cried out, "Help me, I'm hurt!" I chose the path of make believe, and it felt good.

And why is that? My friends sincerely wanted to help me through this hardship. A good one, in fact, took me to lunch to probe why I was being so cold and stoic. "I thought I was your number one," she told me. If I told her how the words "brain injury" made me want to bury my head in the sand, she would have surely comforted me. But I couldn't say that, because giving voice to pain makes it real, and I wasn't ready. Years later, I would learn what a normal psychological response that is. Sniveling into a used tissue on the couch in my therapist's office, it felt like a boulder had been lifted off my shoulders when she told me that "trauma is simply too unbearable to talk about while it's happening."

People removed from trauma metabolize information with a degree of separateness. But when it's you, the experience is so raw, so immediate, you need a shield to protect yourself from further assaults. It's like having a super power, the ability to deflect horror through make believe. With every ninja slice through the air, we avoid the unbearable details the real world asks of us, and so long as we just keep going, nobody can catch up. After a while, though, pretending takes its toll. It's like that nightmare where you are naked in public. You wish someone would throw a blanket on you, or just wake you up.

Once, I was on my way home from the hospital, stopped at a railroad track, waiting for the light. With my Ford Explorer in park, a particular weariness overcame me, and I collapsed, sobbing, behind the wheel. I punched a friend's number, finally ready to share my awful truth—I was scared, and the situation seemed hopeless. "Maggi," I moaned. "Miles weighs 152 pounds." The phone was wet against my cheek. "His skin just hangs off his bones." From her, not a single word about how lucky we'd been. My force field thinned a bit after that. I learned that there are people who will weep with you in silent compassion.

In my experience, survivors and caregivers (who are also survivors), don't seek pity. We march on, managing work projects, coaching soccer, feeding our families. The switch I'm convinced all humans have, dormant until required, flares like an infection the moment we hear the unalterable news that a loved one's life is at risk. We are lit inside, hurt and burning. And yet, it is as Austrian neurologist and

Holocaust survivor Viktor E. Frankl said, "What is to give light must endure burning."

One thing I'd do differently, if I could go back to that meeting with the microphone, is not worry so much about what people think. I'd tell them, when they asked, that my husband suffered damage to his frontal lobe, that he can no longer work as an arborist, and it is likely he will have cognitive limitations. I envision myself, quiet and accepting, as their jaws drop or their eyeballs bulge. My work as caregiver is more important than managing strangers' anxiety. The rest is the same. I'd go to my desk, do my job, go home, and take care of my family.

~Sarah Kishpaugh

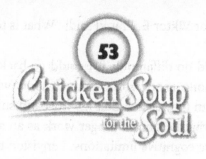

Miracle #2

Gratitude bestows reverence, allowing us to encounter everyday epiphanies, those transcendent moments of awe that change forever how we experience life and the world.
~John Milton

I apprehensively watch from the end of our dead-end road, the book I had been reading long forgotten as my son puts his hand-me-down Ford Escape into reverse. I want to tell him I have a bad feeling about this but he cannot hear me. Just as I think about the SUV skidding out of control, it does. Oh, Lord! This is what I have feared. It's happening again. The distance separating us feels like a great divide. I hear the awful squeal of rubber grinding against loose rocks and hot asphalt. I see a cloud of grey and smell the burn of tires. The book thrown haphazardly on the road, my feet take off running, pounding in time with the refrain "I have to save him, I have to save him."

The SUV disappears completely from my view. I hear a very loud "Boom!" Then, complete and total silence surrounds me. As if from a great distance, I hear myself screaming his name out to the surrounding woods. I feel like I am moving in slow motion, like my feet are stuck in mud. Why am I not getting to him faster? Out of breath, I gasp for air and push myself with every ounce of energy I possess to keep propelling my body onward, lungs burning. I do not want to face what I am about to come upon.

When I arrive, what I see takes away my last remaining breath.

Ugly black scars on the road, leading to what? I collapse upon the road my nose breathing in the hot aroma of heat rising from the street and I think that perhaps I am seeing an apparition. Maybe my mind has finally broken. For standing all in one piece, and outside his totaled SUV, is my son Wesley. While in the background lies his crushed and useless vehicle. A foreign obstacle in this otherwise serene scene: front tires no longer attached, bent metal and shattered windshield, engine still running.

Something is wrong with this picture. Wesley is all in one piece, not lying slumped against the steering wheel as I had envisioned. I look at the mangled SUV and then back at my son, my mind refusing to make the connection. He even appears to be in his right mind because he calls out to me: "Mom?" I look and around see the neighborhood girls come running down the road towards me. I must be in shock. It feels too quiet and surreal. Finally, I spring into action. I want to hug Wesley and reprimand him at the same time. But then I remember he had a passenger.

Jennifer, his girlfriend, where is she? I run through the woods to him and by this time he is helping her through the busted, back passenger side window. He sets her down. She appears all in one piece. But I finally notice all the blood running from their arms and legs from the glass that has pierced their tender flesh. While trying not to give in to my fear, I manage to get them both inside my vehicle and speed away to the nearest medical center.

All the while I am driving with my caution lights flashing, I am reliving the past. This is the same child who survived a traumatic brain injury from a dirt bike accident on this very road on almost exactly this same date years ago. I always dreaded the experience of Wesley getting behind the wheel of a car for the first time. I tried to be extra careful when I finally taught him to drive, and I was very proud of both of us the day we walked into the local DPS office and he got his driver's license. All I could think about was what he had overcome to get to this point in time. But look at us now. "Here we go again," I thought.

Luckily, everything turned out fine for both Wesley and Jennifer.

No head injuries, no broken bones and no stitches. Just sore muscles and a lesson learned and time spent sitting home without something to drive. Wesley was just being a kid that day. A kid who did not think about how his actions behind the wheel of a car could affect the lives of others as well as himself. But luckily he got to have another chance to try it all again. I do not feel that fate stepped in that day. No, I know without a doubt that something unseen was present for Wesley that day just as it has been in his life now for nineteen years. Wesley, you see, has a mission, and until that mission here is accomplished, he will remain and for that I am more grateful than these words on this page can begin to describe.

~Carolyn Hanna Graham

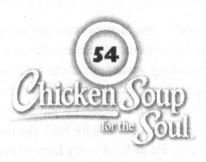

54

Caring About the Adult TBI Survivor

Some of us think holding on makes us strong; but sometimes it is letting go.
~Herman Hesse

My son Neil was seventeen when he sustained a traumatic brain injury at the hands of a drunk driver who hit him and his girlfriend Trista as they were walking. Trista was killed. That was ten years ago. Initially helpless in an intensive care unit, Neil had no choice but to allow his family to take care of him in a way that had not been necessary since he was a small boy. His father carried him to the bathroom. His brother fed him smoothies from a straw. I brushed his unruly curls, massaged his muscles and helped with the exercises his therapist recommended.

Back home, I spotted him like a gymnastics coach as he teetered weakly on his crutches. I made charts for his medication schedule, terrified I would overdose him on pain meds or cause a seizure if I missed an anti-epileptic pill. I kept track of his oral intake and urine output, afraid that he would get dehydrated. Later, I arranged for neuropsychological evaluations, then went to school meetings to advocate for academic modifications based on those results. I drove him back and forth to school, physical therapy and counseling sessions.

At a time in his life when most young people are exerting their independence, moving away from their families and aligning themselves more with peers than parents, my son was thrown back, against his will, to a time of more vulnerability and need. Initially he acquiesced readily, taking advantage of the held hand, the shoulder to lean on, the gripping embrace of family. But eventually he began to bristle at our offers, wanting to rejoin his more independent peers.

College was a constant struggle for Neil. His memory difficulties made academics hard. He utilized every form of extra help available and still just managed to eke out mediocre grades, far less shiny than he was used to. But his social life also suffered from his anxiety and depression. He avoided people, unsure if he knew them. If he did know them, he was unsure of the context, who had introduced them, their names.

Today he is in a better place. Ten years have passed. He is in a Ph.D program for mathematics education. He still suffers from anxiety and sees a therapist from time to time. But he's coping better. He has learned to advocate for himself. He recently petitioned the disabilities office on campus for extra test-taking time and a distraction-free environment. He has a long-term girlfriend, Jen, his first since Trista died.

But I still worry about him. As every parent of adult children knows, they will always be our babies. As the saying goes, "You're only as happy as your saddest child." The brain injury adds a layer of complexity to the angst. I worry about Neil in a way I don't his older brother. I mine each conversation we have for hidden signs of depression or anxiety. With Jen, I have an ally. She sometimes acts as my eyes and ears. When Neil doesn't answer my phone calls, I can text her. When he seems to be having a rough day, she often knows why. She is also my cushion and comfort. Or I should say, Neil's. When we are out at family gatherings—which with our large clan automatically constitutes a crowd, automatically making Neil anxious—she keeps up their end of the conversation long after Neil's hood has come up over his head, long after he's checked out. They hold each other's hands under the table, I can see, each comforting the other.

Caring *for* Neil has morphed into caring *about* him. His girlfriend has taken over as his main source of support. And that is just fine with me.

~Carolyn Roy-Bornstein

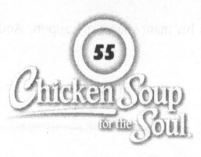

55

The Sounds of Music

A bird doesn't sing because it has an answer. It sings because it has a song.
~Lou Holtz

My dad has always been an impromptu singer and whistler. During any given conversation, he need hear but a word and he will belt out a tune, made up or otherwise, to fit the word he just heard. As a young girl, I remember playing with friends during summer break and hearing a familiar whistle coming from at least a block away; it was my dad, driving toward home, windows down and whistling as loud as he could. Trying to sleep at night, a sudden song would wake me up. Dad was getting ready for bed, and of course, I would whine that he was too loud for me to sleep. Out in public, my dad would start to sing or whistle anywhere or anytime he felt like breaking out in song. How annoying and embarrassing my sister, brother and I thought it was!

One particular day when Dad was singing his best and loudest tune, I asked my mother, "How can you stand listening to Dad's noisy singing and whistling all the time?" She responded, "I think of the day when I will no longer be able to hear it." I thought about my mom's response many times through the years as my dad's voice would fill the world around me, but it wasn't until a few months ago that those words would impact me in a way I never could imagine.

After my grandfather passed away, my dad purchased the family farm where he grew up. Then, a few years after my parents retired, they sold their house of nearly forty years, and moved into the house on the farm. I think no matter where my dad lived, he always considered the farm his "home." It is beautiful there, with tree-filled hills and the constant babble of the creek. It seems that my dad is happiest when he is on the farm puttering in the field or fixing equipment. This is evident when you pull into the drive and see him walking to greet you in his overalls, a smile on his face, belting out a tune.

Now that my parents live on the farm, a two-hour drive away from me, I take every opportunity to see them when they come back to the city for an occasional doctor's visit. One Friday in mid-March my parents were coming to town for such an appointment and we planned to meet for lunch around 11:00 a.m. I'm a night owl, and usually sleep until at least 9:00 a.m. Since many of my friends and family members seem to forget this fact, I tend to turn my phone ringer down or off at night. On this Friday I woke up to find the message light flashing on my phone, not unusual; the message from my mom however was unusual. She and Dad were already in town, and wouldn't meet me for lunch. Dad had slipped on the ice, hit his head and was having emergency brain surgery. Many tears and prayers followed.

I cried out loud as I got dressed, threw on my heaviest winter coat and gloves and rushed off to the hospital. When I arrived, family members and friends were sitting with my mom. As they left one by one, my mom and I were alone; my brother and sister and their families live out of town. Within an hour, although it seemed like an eternity, the surgeon arrived with news that the surgery had gone well; he had removed the blood that had been creating pressure on Dad's brain.

After putting out many prayer requests, and after a couple more hours of waiting, we finally got to see my dad. By then, my brother and one of my nieces had arrived. As we entered the room, we were very delighted to see a man, head wrapped in gauze, neck in a brace, but very alert and very talkative. One of the first things he asked his surgeon was: "Will this affect my singing voice?" Well that was a good sign; the surgeon was very optimistic and he even mentioned the possibility of going home the following Monday. What wonderful news!

Saturday, however, things weren't going quite as planned and on Sunday morning my dad was having a second surgery. Again, I rushed to the hospital, driving with tear-filled eyes, and after many long hours of waiting, news finally came and we were able to see my dad. I was horrified when I first saw him, face swollen, not talking… definitely not thinking about singing. I couldn't stay in the room. The surgeon's words were, in effect, "wait and see."

As the days passed there were slight improvements. Tears filled my eyes as I watched my dad struggle to walk and eat. Finally, after what seemed to be one of the longest weeks of my life, Dad was released to a rehab center. I wasn't sure I agreed that he should be going quite so soon. The next day, as I started down the corridor to my dad's room, I could hear a familiar voice singing in the distance. My dad was singing! I couldn't believe it, nor could I believe my eyes when I first entered the room and saw the father I knew before his fall, except for the many bright blue stitches around his head. More tears, this time tears of joy, and prayers, prayers of thankfulness.

Through it all, my mom's strength amazed me. Through long days spent in the hospital, rarely leaving my dad's side, and the all-day trips to the rehab center, I never once saw her break down. How she kept her composure I'll never know. Three weeks after my dad's fall, thanks to family and friends, prayers and love, my mom was finally able to take my dad home.

Of course there's still healing left for my dad, but one thing that has already healed is his singing and whistling. Today when I hear him singing in public, whistling while getting ready for bed, or singing "just because," it is not an annoyance to me, but a comfort, for I now realize there will be a day when I won't hear it again. But hopefully that day will not come for a very long time.

~Kristen JD Hyde

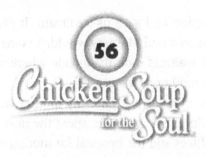

56

My Mom's TBI

To us, family means putting your arms around each other and being there.
~Barbara Bush

My mother has seizures. She was diagnosed when I was ten. Doctors started her on Dilantin immediately. Then began the search for the cause. Questions were hurled at her. The most common was if she had had any brain injuries in the past three, six, or twelve months.

Back then, medical science hadn't realized that a person with a head injury could be at risk for up to fifteen years. My mother had been in an abusive relationship before she met my father. To this day she has a tiny piece of glass embedded in the back of her neck from the abuse.

Her seizures altered our lives. My sister and I were taught the proper steps to take if my mother had one while our father was at work. On our fridge, there were no happy pictures; there was just a list of emergency numbers to call: one for our dad and one for our grandparents. My sister and I took turns sleeping with our mother in case of an attack.

We saw our first seizure a little later in the year. It happened at a very crowded Ryan's. Our mother let out a growl and food began dribbling down her chin. My father nearly upended the table as he caught her before she hit the floor. My sister and I started crying when he leaned her over his lap to keep her from choking.

At that point, a very nice waitress came and took us to the

reserved party section and gave us ice cream. It did little to keep us from crying. I was so afraid Mommy wouldn't come home. About ten minutes later the waitress took us outside where we saw our father half carrying our mother to the car.

An ambulance had arrived, but my mother was very agitated at the thought of riding in it. My mom spent the next few weeks in and out of doctors' offices and the hospital for more tests. Still no cause.

My sister would no longer sleep with my mom in case she had a seizure. She was too frightened. I was the oldest so I did it. God blessed us. We didn't have to deal with a seizure on our own until I was thirteen.

I was sleeping in my own room that night because my father was supposed to be home around 3:00 in the morning. We had just acquired a new puppy that kept me company. It was 1:00 a.m. and I was sleeping soundly. A whining noise from the puppy woke me. The dog was on the floor. I shrugged it off and tried to roll over and drift back to sleep. My arm was hanging off the side of the bed. Katie, the puppy, whined again and sank her little puppy teeth into my arm.

Naturally, I got up and flicked the light on to see how bad the wound was. It wasn't too deep. Then I looked for the dog. She whined from my parents' room. When I looked in, the dog was licking my mother's feet as her body convulsed on the bed. I screamed for my sister.

Carla grabbed the phone and cried when she couldn't reach my father. He was already on his way home and out of cell phone range. She did reach my grandparents. The whole time, she followed my orders and even broke her toe getting things for me.

About seven minutes later my mother came out of her seizure. To our dismay she did not know who we were. I got her to the living room so she would be less inclined to sleep. Her doctor said she should not sleep for two hours after a seizure.

That was when my grandfather showed up. When he entered the house my mother slurred, "Who are you?"

Pawpaw looked at her and said, "Deanna, it's Daddy. Your girls called me." Mom looked around confused and said, "What girls? I don't have any girls." I was reluctant to go back to bed and leave my mom, but I had to go to school the next day.

The next week my mother had a new doctor and a new prescription. Tegratol changed everything for all of us. In the decade since, my mother has had only one seizure. She is now a full-time secretary. Her new doctor wanted to do tests but Mom said she didn't care how she got the seizures. She had them now and she just had to deal with them.

~Brittany Perry

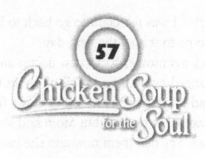

57

The Man Behind the Voice

It is such a secret place, the land of tears.
~Antoine de Saint-Exupéry

I stumble out of bed from a deep sleep to let the dog out during the wee hours of the morning only to discover the light flashing on the answering machine. I press play. "Rick has been in an accident. He has a brain injury. He's in surgery right now. They don't know if he will survive."

I am now wide awake and in shock as to what I should do next. The frightening reality is that my brother might be dying in a hospital four hundred miles away. My brother is having brain surgery. Brain surgery! What can I do?

Speaking with my parents by telephone, I seek solace in the predawn hours. They say the doctor informed them that if Rick survives the operation to remove damaged tissue in his frontal lobe, he will likely have a dull, unemotional personality. Then I call my younger brother Kenny, a truck driver who just two hours earlier had driven through Lubbock. He U-turns his rig and heads back.

As the first rays of light pierce through the darkness of night I call a close friend who lives in Lubbock. Before the devastating news even stumbles from my mouth, Martha interjects, "I'm on my way!" She throws on clothes, a dab of make-up, and rushes out the door.

Two days later my parents and older sister Katrinka arrive at the hospital. Being the self-appointed family historian, I ask Katrinka to take Rick's photo to chronicle his progress. She agrees, but then after seeing him, she rescinds the offer.

Within days, the doctors begin reducing the medications to ease Rick out of his drug-induced coma. He's beginning to respond like someone talking in his sleep. We all wonder: when he is alert, what he will be like? Will he know who we are? Was the doctor correct? Will he have a flat affect?

I am on my way to the hospital. I have a car full of kids and as we approach the outskirts of Lubbock I call Katrinka on her cell phone. She and my parents have been on duty and are ready for relief. Dad is spoon-feeding Rick. He stops to pull Rick upright as he has begun to lean. Rick slurs, "Let go of me, you old fart." The kids hear this and shriek, "He called Granddaddy an old fart!"

The number of visitors in Rick's room is a rule-breaker but we all need a look-see at this rebel who calls his dad an old fart. His eyes are open and we badger the poor guy with questions. "Do you know who I am?"

"My sister," he replies.

Another asks, "Do you know who I am?"

It goes on until he passes the test on each family member.

His eyes track Katrinka like a baby does its mother. She has been his primary caregiver and now it's my turn. As Katrinka, my parents, and the kids prepare to leave, Katrinka says, "I love you, Ricky." He cracks flatly, "I love you, Lucy" and we all scream, "We got Ricky back!" We are thrilled that he is his quick-witted self and is joking about *I Love Lucy*.

We keep a journal on the nightstand. A family member logs what Rick eats or spits out like a baby when he doesn't like his puréed food. We also log the names of visitors. Numerous friends make a two-hour drive to visit. He won't remember these challenging days. Hopefully reading the journal someday will encourage him.

One friend, a man named Roy whom I do not know, phones long distance. I give him the rundown on Rick's progress. Then Roy asks me to put the phone to Rick's ear. And he prays. After several daily calls I immediately recognize the voice on the phone as Roy's and, without fail, he asks that I place the phone to Rick's ear. And he prays.

It's amazing how slowly time passes in a hospital. Finally, Rick is transferred for cognitive rehabilitation. He doesn't remember the early days of hospitalization, nor that he had been at a class reunion and a classmate shoved him. We are all trying to move forward. Four more months away from home is a lonely and fearful time for Rick.

At last, free to return home and independent living, Rick remarks, "Faith is easy to talk about and hard to live." Not quite the jovial prankster and perhaps a bit more serious, he's still the same old Rick to us. We are grateful for his miraculous recovery and elated he will return to his job.

Remembering names of those he meets remains an asset and vital in the sales position he's held for ten years. Eight months after his return, he loses his job. Being fired is a new life experience. He changes careers, passes the real estate licensing exam and loses another position.

I telephone Rick almost daily and I hear the recurring muffled whimper of repressed tears, the uneven breathing. I know he is struggling with depression.

"How can I help?" I ask.

"Just pray," he whispers. He is with it enough to know he's not with it. I am gravely concerned. I ask friends and family to pray for him.

On a crisp October afternoon Kenny telephones. "Rick shot himself."

"God, why did you save him and then let him take his life?" I bawl in agony.

If I had known the high risk of suicide after a TBI, I would have... what? Eventually I must release the "wish I would haves" and "wish I could haves" for my own sanity.

At his funeral, many well-wishers offer condolences. A stranger begins to speak. Before he can introduce himself I smile and say, "I recognize your voice. You must be Roy."

~Belinda Howard Smith

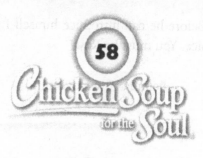

58

Adam

Vitality shows in not only the ability to persist but the ability to start over.
~F. Scott Fitzgerald

I will never forget the neurosurgeon's words: "Please prepare yourself. If he does recover, he won't be quite the same son you knew. No one is ever the same after traumatic brain injury."

Adam struggled through his teenage years. Academically bright but continually frustrated. A typical teen, we thought. We'd had the bleached "Eminem" haircut, the dope-fuelled rebellion and the sudden lunchtime "flu"—distinctly alcohol-related.

What would be next?

As any angst-filled parent of an eighteen-year-old will tell you—it's the car. How would we survive the agonizing years of a teen who can legally drink and legally drive, and perhaps will do both at the same time? I clearly remember the palpable fear that dogged my nighttime hours every weekend.

Unfortunately, my fears were finally realized.

That Saturday night was the perfect storm. It was raining heavily and the roads were wet and treacherous. I was on tenterhooks as Adam drove out of the garage.

"Please be careful," I shouted after him.

"It's Saturday night, Ma." His words hung in the air.

As I went to bed that night I had that sinking feeling in my gut that speed, the weather, alcohol and teen bravado were all conspiring to wreak their havoc. Rog, my husband, was used to my maternal moaning and snored loudly beside me. Then came the phone call. That hospital call will haunt me forever.

There he lay. My big, little boy—so beautiful—and so still. No sign of torment on his innocent face and no sign of the horrific injuries that were yet to manifest themselves as his broken body prepared to struggle for survival.

We were not given any reason to be hopeful by the doctors. We were given many reasons to prepare ourselves for the worst. Most of the bones in Adam's face were broken and his neck was fractured. The impact of the steering wheel smashing into his head as his car swerved off the road and hit a tree at over a hundred kilometers per hour was catastrophic. Thankfully, nobody else had been in the car.

"I'm so sorry. If he does pull through, he'll probably have irreparable brain damage." The doctor's words tore at me.

Rog and Nick, my older son, were my crutches during the zombie-like days to follow. They held me and hugged me as we kept a vigil at Adam's bedside, consumed by fear and heartache as we prayed for our stubborn son's spirit to win his battle for life. He'd survived the eight-hour operation on his face as surgeons meticulously realigned and pinned together his facial bones. But his brain had borne the brunt of the accident, the swelling so great that both sides of his skull had to be removed to allow it to expand.

Hour after hour, we stared numbly at the monitors... beep, beep, beep... waiting, hoping and praying for a miracle. Would the Adam we knew pull through to live, laugh and walk again?

I was very silent in those raw days of deadening grief. I was surrounded by people who cared, really cared. And although well-meaning friends and relatives were constantly in touch, I couldn't face anyone except for my husband and sons. My mum and dad were the exceptions. They kept our family afloat with their stoicism and support. Meals were quietly provided and laundry efficiently dealt with. I could not have endured without my family. We all knew that as long as Adam pulled through, we would be there for him—no matter what.

Then, after the most torturous week... I'm sure I saw his eyes flicker. Maybe his favourite strains of Guns N' Roses had penetrated the comatose days after all? Coming out of a coma is not as it appears in the movies; or at least it wasn't in Adam's case. It was a terrible time of fear and panic and restraining of limbs, which sought to tear out alien tubes. I longed for the day when we could at least remove the pipe from his trachea. Perhaps then he'd be able to eat, drink and maybe even talk. I knew this was asking a lot but silently I hoped against hope anyway.

A month later, it happened. The tubes, screws and nose splint had been removed from his body. All that remained was the neck brace and the bandage protecting his stapled head. He lay there staring blankly, mute and unable to move... but glimmers of light were beginning to dawn.

"Blow me a kiss, Adam," I begged and he did—well he tried.

"Move your right toe, Adam," I persisted, and he did. I was ecstatic.

"He's obeying commands," I shouted in amazement.

"He hasn't done that in years." Rog actually laughed. It felt good to hear that long-absent sound.

We tried to contain our excitement, but this was unmistakable progress and we clung to it and wouldn't let go.

"Adam, hold up four fingers... well done. Okay, now three... yes, fantastic, now two... brilliant... now one."

"You're pushing it Kay," Rog murmured, as we held our breath together.

But then slowly in typically determined Adam style, up came his middle finger. His sense of humour and defiant spirit had won through. The nurses gathered round and we laughed and cried. Never had anyone been so ecstatic to see that gesture! That was the moment I knew Adam—the real Adam—was back.

Slowly he regained his speech, but it took many long, painful patient months of rehabilitation before Adam took his first tentative steps. Wheelchairs, catheters, and physiotherapy filled our days and dominated our lives. I had given up work and spent every waking moment with Adam, only going home to sleep when the hospital bedded down for the night. Even then, I "astral-travelled" to my boy every night, willing him on:

"I know you can do this. You've never given up on anything."

I remember Adam's homecoming clearly. It had taken five months to live a lifetime. "Drive carefully. We're nearly there," I cautioned Rog, as we left the hospital with our precious passenger. There were still many hurdles to cross but we were ready to tackle the future again. Adam's memory had blanked out the accident itself but he was fully aware of everything else, and he knew he had been given a second chance.

"It's good to be home, Ma," he smiled.

He didn't blow that chance. He is now coming to the end of his double-degree in law and behavioural science, and he's met a wonderful partner with whom he wants to share his life. He's still not ready to drive and he has some peripheral vision impairment, but I can honestly say that my beautiful, strong boy is the Adam I know.

There were many times during that desperate journey when hopelessness and despair almost overwhelmed me, and hope and prayer were all I clung to. But as horrific as the experience was, I learned that traumatic brain injury is not always the end. It can also be a new beginning.

~Kay Ward

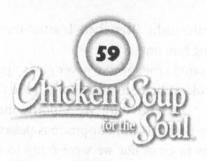

59

The Problem with a Miracle

War does not determine who is right — only who is left.
~Bertrand Russell

The problem with a miracle is that you want to be grateful all the time but sometimes that can be hard. On April 28, 1970, Allen walked away from a devastating plane crash in Vietnam, injured but alive. It was a miracle. But miracles can be challenging, especially those that involve a burning plane and the man you love.

Of course it's easy to be grateful when we're with our children celebrating the great and small moments of family life and I remember his six crewmates who didn't survive, or when we settle on the sofa to watch a movie, or when the engine warning light comes on in the car and I hand it off to him to handle, and especially when he wraps his arms around me and just breathes.

But then, it's harder to be grateful when he gets depressed and sleeps for days, or clings to me when I want some time to myself, and especially, when he becomes someone I don't know, when anger takes over a piece of him.

After the crash, his skin healed, with a few visible scars, and I thought he was fine. But there was internal injury. We didn't know about that, or how it would change him in unexpected ways at unexpected times for unexplainable reasons. Now we know he has a traumatic brain injury. He escaped the flames, but they kept consuming him. As he's gotten older, the brain trauma is fueled by post-war demons, and sometimes I feel like I am losing him to that burning plane after all.

Before the crash Allen was an easygoing, cheerful, kind, gentle guy who told silly jokes and thought they were hilarious. After the crash, he was just the same. It was amazing! No nightmares. No fears. He even flew on planes when our trips to visit family were too far away to drive. He talked about the crash if someone was interested, but otherwise didn't dwell on it too much. Clearly, the psychologists who treated him after the crash had done a great job.

I eased into life with Allen like a pair of jeans that gets more comfortable over time, until they become your favorites. Really, comfy well-worn jeans you can depend on to feel right every time you put them on—now that's a long-term relationship.

The thing is, those favorite jeans can get worn in places, and eventually a hole appears. A marriage is like that. Over time, some places get too comfortable and the next thing you know, they're worn through. Then there's a decision to make. I can throw out the jeans or I can patch the hole. I think it's better to patch the hole, but I know the jeans won't be the same. They'll feel different and I'll have to get used to them, get comfortable in a different way, and once I do, they'll be my favorites again. Being married to someone with traumatic brain injury has meant applying a lot of patches and fixing a lot of holes to find our comfortable place again.

For the first thirty-five years of our marriage, patching the holes worked just fine. But then, the fabric of our relationship started to fray and tear and I just couldn't keep up with all the patching and fixing. Allen tried too, but even together, we just couldn't do it. There were more and more instances when he lost his temper over small things. It was never about us—his family. It was always something related to someone not doing their job right—the waiter getting the order wrong, or the salesman not waiting on the next person in line, and when he got on the phone with the cable TV people, I had to leave the room. It was irrational, embarrassing and even a little frightening. When I tried to talk to him about it, he was annoyed and cut me off.

"It's not about you," he'd snap.

"But it affects me," I'd implore.

"I don't want to discuss it."

Eventually, even Allen recognized that something was breaking down inside him. Ironically, or perhaps predictably, the worst moment happened at the airport. We were flying home from Las Vegas to Chicago with our nine-year-old granddaughter. As we went through the security line, she spotted the sign about removing shoes and said, "They don't have any of those slipper things and I don't have socks on. I don't want to walk through there barefoot." In Chicago's O'Hare airport, there were paper booties to slip on when you took off your shoes, but Las Vegas didn't offer that amenity.

"Sorry, sweetie," I replied. "We'll walk really fast." She was clearly distressed.

Allen stopped a TSA agent, and pointing to our granddaughter's sandals asked, "Does she have to take those off?"

"No, she can leave them on," was the reply. Our granddaughter was happy and we all moved forward. As we got to the front though, a different TSA agent told us to remove our shoes, including our granddaughter, and when we explained that the other agent said she could keep them on, we were told that no, she would have to remove her shoes.

Allen blew up. He started yelling about how people should know their jobs and know what they were telling people and I don't even know what else he was hollering. I tried to get him to calm down, worried he'd be arrested. He shrugged me off. I was horrified for him, for me, and for our granddaughter, who by then had gone through security barefoot and was on the other side. I quickly joined her, tried once again to get Allen's attention, and when he yelled at me to leave him alone, I told him we'd see him at the gate and I took her off to the airport shops. We didn't see him again until just before we boarded the plane. We didn't speak during the entire flight home.

When we got home, he agreed to go to the local Veterans

Administration Hospital and get some help. That was the best decision we could have made. From that point forward, things steadily improved. After a few years of individual and group therapy, and some medication, he got better. It was slow and there were some moments of serious reflection as we came to terms with the reality of an eighty percent disability diagnosis. In fact, he reached a point where the VA sessions were setting him back, actually rekindling some of the anger. He saw other veterans struggling and it was hard for him to be there. So now he sees a private therapist and that has been a helpful transition.

It's still not perfect, but what relationship is? We're still patching holes, finding our comfortable place. Some days it's harder to be grateful than others. But the important thing is, Allen is enjoying life again, we're looking ahead to our retirement years together, and he's much more like the man I fell in love with—an easygoing, cheerful, kind, gentle guy who tells silly jokes and thinks they're hilarious.

~Barbara Chandler

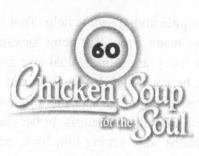

60

A Quiet Night in Mexico

It takes two men to make one brother.
~Israel Zangwill

My mother, father and I sat for a very long time, mostly abstaining from conversation and food, avoiding eye contact. We chewed on the silence, picking its sharp bones from our teeth. An entire meal with only the sound of boards bending and creaking in the winter cold, of clearing throats, of crickets chirping, and of forks scraping against plates as they rearranged small piles of spaghetti; those millions of sounds you notice when there is nothing you can say.

I noticed that maybe a dozen cookbooks were scattered across the kitchen counters, books with the names of countries I'd never been to printed on their covers. Most nights, the smell of seared monkfish or steaming moussaka wafted out of the kitchen accompanied by loud jazz music and my mother's singing if she thought no one was listening. Tonight she served undercooked spaghetti with store-bought pasta sauce and scooped small forkfuls into her mouth. She seemed to forget that the pit in her stomach did not allow room for things like food.

My father managed to force down a few mouthfuls, then pulled his cheeks up in a fake smile, making his jaw labor hard enough that I could almost hear it tremble and groan, like an old wooden bridge sagging under its own damp weight.

I sat with one hand resting on my knee under the table, hiding the not-yet-healed cuts across my knuckles. I could never stop picking at the scabs. My mother was looking at me, waiting for me to force down even one bite, but I just kept pushing around my heap of undercooked pasta until it got cold and I could dump it in the trash, go to my brother's room and just sit—maybe hit play on his CD player and blast whatever was in there.

My brother was in a hospital fifty miles away, living on clear fluid from a tube stuck in his arm. Every hour or so his eyes would start fluttering and he would moan louder and louder until a nurse came into the room and pushed a button, quieting him for a while longer with a push of some drug I couldn't name. A hospital blanket, stiff and uncomfortable, hid his broken and scarred leg. Nothing covered his fractured skull.

A doctor who would forget my brother's name as soon as he took off his stethoscope had come into the room with his Latex-gloved hands clasped on my brother's thin shoulder and told us that there was nothing they could do about the swelling in his brain. It felt to me like they were telling us that all they could do was wrap a line of crime scene tape around it and tell everyone to stand back.

"Right now, you just need to be patient."

I could have killed him. But instead I nodded and said thank you.

He peeled off the Latex gloves and threw them in the trash before he left the room, as if he didn't want to carry our despair into the hallway with him.

My brother looked as if he might only be asleep, but periodically he flailed as much as his body could muster, maybe fighting through broken dreams of shattered glass and screeching tires.

A tear fell from my mother's cheek into her spaghetti. My father didn't move to lay an arm over her shoulder; he never said that everything was going to be all right and not to worry, and it wouldn't have been right if he did. Why even open our mouths? We had all been there when the doctor said; "He might not make it out of this without some brain damage."

Just two days before, I had stepped off a plane to be picked up by my father and brought to the Brigham and Women's Hospital in Boston, Massachusetts. The day before that, I had talked to my mother from a pay phone by the side of the road in Cuernavaca, Mexico.

I can't really remember what my mother said to me that night because I was in shock. A boy walks his girlfriend home just a few nights after Christmas, holding her hand, down a well-lit street. So well lit that neither of them see their shadows cast in front of them, as the screaming headlights of the cherry-red killer bears down on them. The boy now lay in a coma, and the girlfriend's family was hoping they would be able to have an open casket funeral.

I remember the last three words my mother said to me: "Are you okay?" Her question was honest and so was my answer. I slammed the phone down into its cradle.

Again and again, harder each time. I wanted to feel something being destroyed in my hands, even if it was a public telephone in a poor Mexican city. I walked around for hours, a crazy American kid bleeding from the cuts in his hands and stumbling around on a quiet night in a foreign city.

My mother picked up my plate and used her fork to scrape the heap of cold spaghetti onto the pile of her own scarcely touched food along with my father's, an entire empty meal consumed by the garbage disposal in a few short seconds.

We left for the hospital after my mother did the dishes and later that night it rained, washing away the other sounds of the night like patches of blood and bone fragments.

My brother's leg eventually healed and the swelling subsided in his brain. He would mention the accident very rarely. On one occasion, he told me about the final conversation he had with his girlfriend. He said they were walking hand in hand down that well lit street, talking generally about the future. That they no longer spoke in terms of if's but of when's. When I hear him talk now, I know his leg is still broken somewhere and his skull is still fractured, and at night he'll have to curl up in uncomfortable hospital blankets. And I think about how vastly the if's in our lives outnumber the when's, how chance plays a much greater role than we might like to think. And I think about how, even when chance drives through and devastates some of the things we might have been secure about the moment before it happens, there is a glue, a tougher-than-chance rock that we should all be so lucky to have. And that is the love of our family and friends and the people around us whose support makes our lives and the small world we live in better and brighter.

~Dan Bornstein

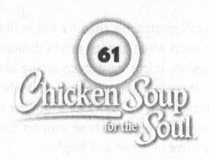

61

Project DownRange

The cruelest lies are often told in silence.
~Adlai Stevenson

We were two weeks away from Christmas and a divorce. My husband was an American veteran, proudly serving in Operation Iraqi Freedom from 2003-2004 when he sustained a traumatic brain injury. If either of us had known about that diagnosis, it might have saved us both a lot of heartache. But that information was not passed along to me, his next of kin, and my husband thought the appointments he had been faithfully going to were simply to help treat his post-traumatic stress disorder.

During the eight years since his return from service, my husband had turned into a man I did not know. Once my beloved high-school sweetheart, he was now the spouse who told me eight times in one year to move out. Something told me I should stay.

My husband one day asked me to go into our safe and retrieve his military health records. Before I handed them over to my husband, I gave the documents a perusal of my own. There, right at the top of the twenty-page file, was his diagnosis from November 2007: "Traumatic Brain Injury. Post-concussion Syndrome."

Because I had some medical background, I understood exactly what those words meant. The anger. The personality changes. The inappropriate behavior. It all suddenly made sense. At that moment I realized that the myriad health issues we had been dealing with for years were attributable to a TBI. It wasn't that my husband no longer loved me like I once thought. It was that his TBI was changing him in ways I hadn't understood before.

Now, two years later, we live on five acres, away from the triggers of the impact zone. I am now able to take care of the needs of our family without the stress of the unknown. Learning not to respond to his unfiltered comments was hard. Some days were harder. Reminding myself that none of us asked for this helps ease the daily struggles. Finding peace within myself during the silence of the day is how I find my inner strength. I am far from perfect but our family is strong enough to survive the battles of brain injuries. Our daughters are understanding when their father's symptoms are heightened and they are compassionate about his memory issues, fatigue and other frustrating symptoms.

This injury might be a hidden wound of war, but in our family it is far from hidden. But it will not define us. In fact, it will only make us stronger. And that's why I started Project DownRange to help educate other military families about the existence of TBIs in their returning heroes.

~Sarah Jenkins

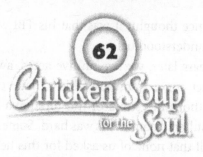

62

Jonathan's Story

Autumn is a second spring when every leaf is a flower.
~Albert Camus

"Please God no, please God no!" I found myself saying over and over in my head, as I ran as fast as I could toward the end of our street. Seconds before, the frantic ringing of the front doorbell had broken the usual tranquility of a Sunday afternoon. As I approached the door, I could hear a panic-filled voice calling out my name. I felt a sudden rush of anxiety, yet I was still unprepared for the terrified appearance of our eleven-year-old neighbour Josh, with his arms flailing about, eyes wide with shock and voice almost hysterical, screaming, "Cheryl—come quick! Jono's been hit by a car!"

"What?" I cried out in disbelief. "Where, Josh? What happened?"

I didn't even wait for his reply, but instead ran out the door and straight past Josh, leaving my son Chris still inside watching television, and the Mexican dinner I had been cooking still simmering on the stove. As I approached the corner of our street I remember thinking to myself, "Why can't I hear him crying? He should be crying!"

It was then that I saw my husband Robert. With a look of sheer torture and panic drawn on his face, a look forever etched in my mind, his hands were held above his head as he ran into the house on the corner of our street, screaming, "Help me, help me! Ring an ambulance!"

It was a Sunday, a lovely autumn Sunday, with amber leaves

strewn across the lawns of the well-kept houses on our street. A day spent at home doing normal family things, Sunday things, together things. Jonathan, then age twelve, had spent most of the day playing outside in the mild warmth of the fall sun with his brother Chris, aged ten, and their friend Josh. They very rarely ventured past the corner of the street, and if they did, they knew to let me know first.

"Mum," Jonathan had said only hours earlier in his husky confident tone as he munched on a toasted sandwich, "I love days like this, when we don't do anything, or go anywhere, just stay home all day. They're my favourite days!"

Simple words, yet ironically they could have been his last.

I kept on running and finally saw my darling boy, my precious Jonathan, lying crumpled like a rag doll on the road. As I knelt down beside him, I knew straight away it was very, very serious. There was an enormous amount of thick, dark-red blood oozing from his nose and mouth. He was on his right side and his eyes were open. I stroked his face and spoke softly to him. Something inside me told me to be calm and not to cry, though every fibre of my being was trembling with fear. I tenderly picked up his limp right hand and said, "Mummy's here darling. You're going to be all right. Just keep breathing. That's right, in and out, nice and slow. Good boy. Just keep breathing. That's right, my baby, you must keep breathing. Don't stop, darling."

I held his hand and kept speaking to him, silently praying for the sounds of an ambulance siren. I knew he could hear me, even though he lay deathly still; his eyes were telling me so. He kept breathing steadily for a few minutes, but then suddenly he vomited. It was then that I began to get truly frightened because his breathing became laboured and his eyes glazed over. I knew I was losing him! I stood up and asked if anyone from the circle of people who had now gathered around us knew CPR. A sea of faces stared back at me, some in horror, others in pity. And then, just as I was about to lose my sanity and scream in desperate fear of what was about to happen, by the grace of God, I heard a siren. I turned and looked down the street and saw the approach of bright flashing lights, standing out against the backdrop of the golden glow of the sunset. For some reason I shall never forget this sunset and the ominous feel it had—it was as if it could be setting on our lives forever....

That was sixteen years ago, but when I go there in my mind, it feels like yesterday. In May 1997, my beautiful boy, who could play three musical instruments, run like the wind, and was at the top of his class academically, was hit by a car whilst crossing the road to come home. Initially he had a Glasgow Coma Score (GCS) of 3 and we were told many times over the ensuing three weeks in intensive care not to expect him to live through the night. He was in a coma for approximately six weeks and had post-traumatic amnesia (PTA) for about ten months. We were told he might never walk, talk or even eat again. But due to his relentless drive and a well-coordinated holistic programme of rehabilitation, he has defied the odds—going back to school to get his high school certificate, working, and even learning to drive. Not only can he walk independently but he can run! He plays tennis, swims laps, plays the piano and snow skis!

Learning that your loved one has suffered a traumatic brain injury is extremely difficult. When you first emerge from the devastating shock and enraged denial, the real pain and heartache are enough to threaten your very existence, and if you let it, the resentment can destroy your soul. The loss of your life as it once was, and the partial loss of the very essence of your loved one, is very, very significant. What can you do? You have only two choices: you can spend your life mourning the fact that your dreams are now shattered, or you can do whatever is within your power and capability to change what can be changed, without forsaking the insight to accept what cannot.

Our family was able to carry on by taking one day at a time and looking to find something positive from each day. The fact that we still had Jonathan in our lives was the main source from which we drew our strength. Even now we still find it best to live our lives one day at a time, enabling us to concentrate on small pleasures; things that in a normal life would be taken for granted, now add richness and colour to our lives. Even though the past decade has been physically demanding and an emotional roller coaster ride, caring for

Jonathan and his ever-changing needs has brought us closer together as a family and enriched our lives in many unexpected ways.

For despite living in a society that values status, production and competition, Jonathan has—through boundless courage and true dignity—taught us that personal credibility doesn't come in the form of I.Q. numbers, degrees or sporting trophies. He has revealed the importance of validating and accepting individuals for who they are and whatever contribution they make to society. He has learnt to not only live with his residual impairments, but to teach those around him to do the same.

Some of the life lessons I've learnt over the last sixteen years are:

- The importance of never giving up hope despite, or perhaps in spite of, foreboding predictions.
- The importance of centering your life on what it is you have—not what you lack.
- The importance of family, friends, and community support.
- The importance of not allowing the barriers other people create to get in the way of what you really want to achieve—never let someone else's doubts blur your vision.

But by far, of all the knowledge I have gained during our journey of hope, discovery and healing, one important fact stands out: recovery cannot be accurately determined by science, nor can potential be predicted, or spirit measured.

~Cheryl Koenig, OAM

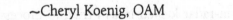

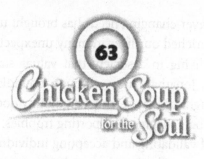

63

Chicken Soup for the Soul

Mind Your Words

Patience and diligence, like faith, remove mountains.
~William Penn

"I'm so sorry," I whispered to my friend as my phone rang again. It was ten-thirty at night and we'd just put her son to sleep. I had already talked to my husband Nathan a half hour before, so why was he calling again?

I slipped into a room furthest from the bedroom and answered quietly, "What do you need, babe? Everyone is asleep."

"Where are you? Why aren't you here?"

I pulled the phone away from my ear to soften the yelling. Was this a joke? Was he angry about something? "I don't even know what you're saying. It's too late to joke around. What's up?"

"I want to know where you are. And where am I? Something is wrong. Something is very wrong and I'm scared."

My mom-radar kicked in as I tried to process his words. If he wasn't joking, then where were the kids? Where was he? I tried to calm him down and get the answers, but I couldn't. He went into hysterics and said his head was bleeding. I was two hours from home and didn't have a clue what was going on. I finally convinced him to put my oldest son—who was nine—on the phone. Adrenaline kicked in as I listened to the role reversal on the other end of the line—my son parenting his father, trying to convince him to sit down and relax. My son trying to reassure me. My son asking if he was supposed to call the cops.

The two-hour drive home was torture. Nathan was Life Flighted out of our home. My children went to a neighbor's and I headed to the University of Virginia's hospital. That night commenced a journey that would consume the next two years of our lives, and then leave traces of change even today.

What I found out was that my husband tripped over a jar left on the basement stairs. His head slammed into an exposed metal corner and a stud on the way down. The police officers who had responded to his accident had seen a similar fall just a year prior, except that victim had been found dead. My husband was very much alive, but incredibly confused about his existence.

A few days after his accident he was sent home with the diagnosis of a traumatic brain injury and a sheet of paper that was supposed to equip us for the next phase of life. It said:

Personality changes are possible.
Memory retention is difficult.
Patient may speak exactly what is on his or her mind.
Sleep patterns will change and insomnia may occur.
Headaches of varying degrees can be expected.
Symptoms may last between twelve and sixty months.

Nathan is a pastor and his office was currently at home. This was a blessing for his work and rest routine, but incredibly difficult on our marriage.

When he slept, he awoke with splitting headaches. He spent hours each day alone in the bedroom with the curtains drawn. Before his fall, he was the fun parent—the one who got the kids all riled up before dinner and wrestled on the carpet with them before bed. After the fall, he would yell downstairs about the noise and how it exacerbated the pain in his head.

When he finally started driving again, he called one day to ask me where he was. He had been on his way home from town, stopped at a stop sign, and forgot which direction he was supposed to be going. Nothing was familiar. He wasn't even sure if he was still in Charlottesville.

Work situations that would normally stress him out suddenly sent him over the edge. He struggled with severe depression. One evening, I found him in the kitchen with a knife, sobbing because he didn't want to live like this. Another time he called me from the road, desperate for me to talk some sense into him; all he wanted to do was to drive his car into a tree and make the pain stop.

And while these situations were intense and demanding, they were nothing compared to the new style of communication which entered our marriage following Nathan's brain injury.

We were upstairs one afternoon, folding laundry together, when something small set us both to arguing. Before the injury, I was the hot-tempered spouse. My past was rough, and often I'd find myself spewing toxic words with the intent of harming my husband. He was always the one who watched what he said. Before the fall, he might match me in volume, but never in volatility. However, on this afternoon, I was forced to accept the fact that my husband as I once knew him might not be the husband standing before me.

I approached the argument in my normal manner, with a lot of words and logical reasoning which were intended to back Nathan into a corner. As I spoke, my husband's hands pressed against his temples, but I didn't stop. I kept right on "reasoning." Suddenly he exploded. "You b—!" he yelled. "You've been driving me crazy for years. Can you please stop talking? I can't stand it anymore. I haven't been able to stand you since before we married."

I did exactly as he asked and stopped talking. Never in my life had I heard him speak like this *about* anyone, much less *to* anyone, and never to me. Who was this man?

I raced down the stairs and out to the car. I hadn't even made it a quarter mile when the Lord had me pull over and look into a mirror.

This, my child, is why you must learn to tame your own tongue. He lashed out at you once, as his brain fights to heal and restore and make new connections. How many times have you lashed out at him over the years?

My husband's words reflected my own illness that had permeated our marriage long before his fall. I turned the car around and went back home. While Nathan's injury continued to affect his personality for the next eighteen months, I resolved to still my tongue and began to practice the art of responding in an argument rather than reacting.

Today, he continues to have headaches and still fatigues easily. By the end of the day he is not in the mood for chaos and noise (which in a family of seven is almost guaranteed), but he has returned to being the encouraging and loving man I married. He is my biggest cheerleader — the same as he was before his accident — and I am his, which is where the real healing has been found.

~Marian Green

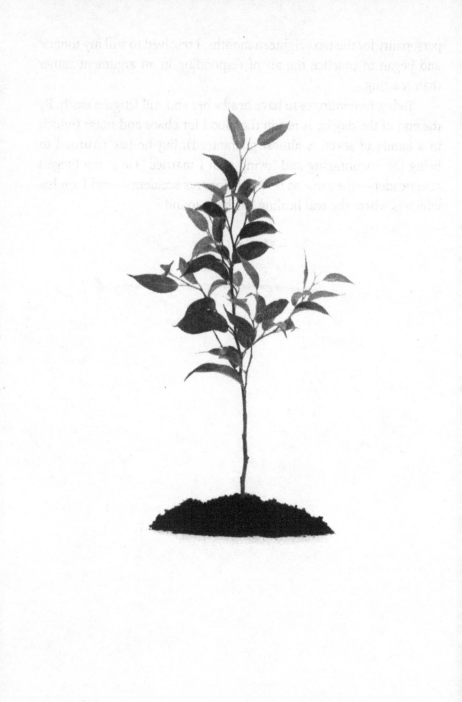

Chapter 7

Recovering *from* Traumatic Brain Injuries

Attitude Is Everything

Chapter

7

Recovering from Traumatic Brain Injuries

Attitude Is Everything

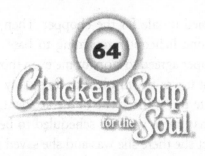

64

HollyDay Miracles

There are only two ways to live your life. One is as though nothing is a
miracle. The other is as though everything is a miracle.
~Albert Einstein

I've been called an overachiever since I was a very little girl, but it's only in the last year or two that I have come to realize that the label may actually fit me. I have always believed that anything worth doing is worth doing well, and so I have always tried to do my best at all times no matter what the task at hand might be. Who knew that this ingrained philosophy would one day save my life?

I was a twenty-one-year-old college senior just beginning my student-teaching internship instructing high school students in vocal music. Eager to share my love of music with these young people, I was undaunted by the long drive home that day in a torrential downpour. The winding, hilly country road was flooding, but there I was feeling on top of the world and looking forward to writing my lesson plans for the next day's classes. The next thing I knew, I awoke in a hospital three months later.

I was told that I'd been in a two-car collision but that I'd been the only one physically injured in the crash. I was also told that I owed my life to a series of miracles, the first one being the arrival of a nurse on the scene who proceeded to climb into my mangled car with me and hold me tight as we waited for the help to arrive that she had summoned. This angel-nurse then insisted that I be flown to the hospital via helicopter, even though the weather was so foul that it had been deemed unsafe for the chopper. Then, another miracle. There was only one helicopter returning to base that was still airborne. That chopper agreed to stop for me even though the pilot had been warned that it was not prudent to do so. My angel-nurse then helped to intubate me at the scene of the accident, as I was already unresponsive. That nurse was not scheduled to be on that road, at that hour, and yet she there she was and she saved my life.

Since that night, I have been surrounded and lifted up by more miracles than I can recount here. One is the fact that, although I suffered eleven broken bones from the accident (two femurs, one hip, one tibia, one humerus, one vertebra and five ribs) I never felt any pain at all because they all healed during the three months I lay unresponsive in a coma. I survived several bouts of infection in those limbs as well—perhaps another miracle! Maybe the greatest miracle of all is the continuous recovery I am still having after sustaining such a serious traumatic brain injury. Known as a diffuse axonal injury, it affected every area of my brain, yet I have confounded several doctors and therapists as I have continually healed above and beyond their expectations. My healing has been and continues to be a miracle.

They say that everything happens for a reason, so I have to wonder if my accident was a part of some great cosmic plan for my life! Maybe the reason I was always so driven to succeed through hard work was to prepare me for this—the greatest challenge of my life. Because I was always so driven in my studies, I had accumulated four years' worth of college credits in just three years, enough to graduate with my class, on time, with honors, and just eight months after the accident. Now there's a real miracle!

My family and I have been the recipients of so many acts of kindness since the accident that we could never repay: all of the family, friends, coworkers, acquaintances and total strangers who have guided us, supported us and just plain loved us as we made our way through the weeks and months of recovery. The circle of care surrounding us has been one of our best miracles. New friendships have been forged and our circle of love is still widening to this day. To me, it's a miracle that I finally feel understood and appreciated, even a little vindicated in my early overachieving days!

I am twenty-three years old now and we will soon celebrate the second anniversary of my accident. I've named the day after myself. I call it "HollyDay." It's a celebration of the miracle of my continued existence on this planet. I am still healing and continue outpatient therapies three days per week. I also volunteer in my community and am about to take a college class in preparation for future graduate level work. I am considering a change in my career path, but this is still uncertain at this time. What is certain is that I have benefited from a long string of miracles—and I am grateful.

~Holly Daubenspeck

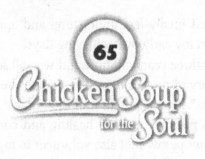

65

Back on Top of the World

A goal is a dream with a deadline.
~Napoleon Hill

I was on top of the world. I was twenty-four, dating a terrific guy, and had just been hired as a middle school band director, my dream job. I was already involved with summer marching band and excited about what the year would bring.

I was leaving an evening marching band rehearsal when I made a left turn from a stop sign directly in front of a 17-ton Mack truck that hit my driver's side door going fifty-five miles per hour. I have no memory of the accident or the month that followed.

My parents kept their hopes up that I would get better. I had been in a coma for days and the doctors couldn't explain why I wasn't waking up. They talked to my parents about institutionalizing me. My accident was on August 13th. My dad's birthday is August 20th. During those days he would tell me his birthday was coming and that I needed to open my eyes: "My birthday is in four days. All I want is for you to open your eyes." Then Mom would say, "Dad's birthday is in two days. All he wants is for you to open your eyes." When the day arrived, Dad took my hand and said, "Chris, today is my birthday and all I want for my birthday is for you to open your eyes. Please open your eyes." I did, briefly. They ran to share the news with my doctor, who downplayed it, telling them that it was simply a coincidence. In my heart, I know I did it deliberately.

I drifted in and out of consciousness. My cognition at that time was very fuzzy. I thought all the tubes sticking out of my arms were snakes. I had to be restrained to keep from pulling them out. I had four stable breaks in my pelvis. My parents didn't mention the traumatic brain injury I suffered because they were afraid it would discourage me. Eventually I figured this out on my own when I couldn't read the items around me.

I eventually learned how close I came to death that first night. The fire department, which cut my car apart with two sets of the Jaws of Life, called the hospital the next morning to check on my status. They were told that I had made it through the night, but would likely die in the next few hours.

The predictions were so negative! I wouldn't live through the first twenty-four hours. I would never regain consciousness. I would be greatly diminished cognitively. I would have a different personality. I would never walk or drive again. There was only a fifty percent chance that I would return to teaching in six or seven years. But every prediction the doctors made proved wrong.

I was ranked a 4 on the Glasgow Coma Scale. This scale goes from 3-15. Scoring a 3 means that the patient is totally non-responsive. Four is a very bad rating. Years later when I spoke at a music therapy conference, my parents talked to the doctor on the panel about how frustrating it was to have the doctors constantly dash their hopes for my recovery. He explained, "Ninety-eight percent of those who score a 4 on the Glasgow Scale don't get better. It really is a miracle!"

My cognitive abilities improved with therapy. A nurse asked me what college I attended. I told her. Her response was, "That's an expensive school!"

I replied, "It is, but I had a…" I couldn't come up with the word and she wasn't going to help me. Frustrated I asked, "What's it called when they give you the money?" She smiled. "A scholarship!"

She saw the look on my face and explained, "You just made a

new neural connection. The word was there all the time. The old pathway was destroyed, but you just made a new pathway!"

The same thing happened when I relearned my clarinet. Occasionally I would have to be reminded of a note name, term, or fingering. I only needed to hear it once and it was re-established in my mind. It was frustrating to not know when knowledge would be missing, but a relief to know that it could be relearned.

Two things happened that made a tremendous impact upon my recovery. First, I overheard the doctor tell my mother that he wasn't sure I would walk again. I prayed to God, "Please help me to walk. I'll do the work, whatever needs to be done." Second, during therapy to stretch my bent arm, a therapist asked me to put a ball in the box with my left hand. I couldn't move my arm at all. I finally pulled the box forward with my right hand and dropped the ball in with my bent left arm. The therapist was mad.

Suddenly I realized what needed to be done. I asked, "What's the objective? What's the *real* objective?" The teacher in me understood that surface goals were being used for a greater purpose. She explained that she was trying to stretch my arm out. I replied that after being in so much pain, I was going to find the least painful way to accomplish the surface goal presented to me. She told me, "If you want to get better, it's going to hurt." After that conversation, she told me the real goal. I forged on through the pain to meet those goals. My recovery took off.

The day I was admitted to the rehabilitation hospital, tents were set up outside. My parents learned that a survivors' picnic is held each year to celebrate those who recover. They told the staff that we would return as survivors the next year. The following year at the picnic, the staff shared the story of my recovery before presenting me with the Phoenix Award for the year's most remarkable recovery. Like the phoenix, I had returned to life from the ashes of death.

The story doesn't end there. I eventually got my life back. I had the same personality. I could walk and drive. I returned to teaching the next fall and started school to earn my master's degree the year after that. I married my boyfriend, who had the courage to see me through this, and we have a beautiful daughter. I'm once again on top of the world.

~Christine R. Blue

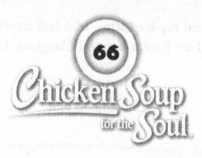

66

How I Learned to Walk

Growth is an erratic forward movement: two steps forward, one step back.
Remember that and be very gentle with yourself.
~Julia Cameron

I have always been lucky—very lucky. I was twenty-five, I had a great factory job, and I had won back my childhood sweetheart. Linda was beautiful, inside and out, with a quick and curious mind. She also had a great job working for the city. In 1988 we bought a house, got engaged, and had set our wedding date for June 24, 1989.

On January 26th of that same year, I pulled out in front of a semi-truck on my way home from work. I don't remember this; I don't really remember most of the 1980's. Everything I know about that day has been told to me by other people. The volunteer EMTs that responded to the call were all friends of mine from work, and what I know about what happened to me that day I gathered from them. Seeing the crumpled wreckage of my pick-up truck, they at first thought that I must surely be dead. Instead, they found me lying across the seat with barely a pulse. Luckily, the local volunteer rescue squad had received a pneumatic splint less than a month earlier. Without it, they would not have been able to keep my blood pressure sufficiently elevated to keep me alive for the twenty-five minute ambulance ride to the nearest level one trauma center, now called Regions Hospital.

I was diagnosed with a traumatic brain injury—a severe coup-contra-coup type—the equivalent of putting a delicate stereo component in a paint shaker and turning it on for a few minutes. I spent the next ten days in a coma. My body temperature had spiked to over 108 degrees on a couple of occasions and the doctors said it was likely that I had suffered further severe brain damage from that. They told my family to start looking into long-term care facilities or nursing homes. There really is no way to tell the effects of brain injury with any certainty ahead of time; it would be easier to tell what the weather was going to be like a few months out.

As I drifted out of my coma the collectively held breath of my friends and family was allowed to escape. I actually made pretty good progress over the next few weeks; I was starting to remember people's names and even regaining my sense of humor. Late in February, Linda asked me if I wanted to go through with the wedding. We were, after all, planning a big affair with 200 guests, and she needed to know if she should keep planning everything and reserving facilities and the caterer and so forth. I couldn't believe my luck! Here I was in the hospital. I couldn't walk. I could barely talk. I couldn't really dress or bathe myself. And yet the most beautiful and amazing woman I had ever known still wanted to marry me! I said, "Yes, of course."

Well, this was wonderful, but what could I bring to the table? I couldn't bear the thought of her burdening herself with me. I now felt a huge obligation; what could I do to shore up my end of the bargain? I decided that at the very least, I would walk my new wife up the aisle at the end of our ceremony. I would walk by Linda's side, as though she had an equal partner. I would learn to walk. She might have to work full-time, take care of a house, take care of me, and plan a wedding for 200 guests, but I was determined to walk side by side with my bride. I wanted to tell Linda how much I loved her, but my speech was so bad I was embarrassed to say it. I inwardly decided that I would express my love for her by walking. Each step was me saying, "I love you." This was my own resolve, I told no one of my plan.

It may sound simple, but achieving that goal was no small feat. Until that point, I had only taken a few steps, and even then, a nurse was holding me up. On my first day at rehab, a physical therapist wheeled me up to the parallel bars. I stood up and thought, "I love you." I wobbled, but I held my grip. White-knuckled and taking short rapid breaths, I felt like a ski jumper who had just left the ramp. I was only standing, but I felt like I was flying.

"You're doing well, Michael. If you need to sit, just let me know," encouraged the nurse.

I kept going. My legs felt full of water, dull and heavy. Center of balance was a misnomer to me; my balance was anywhere but center. I felt like there was a legion of Lilliputians pulling and tugging at their ropes drawing me to and fro. What I really needed to do was focus, but focus and brain injury are antonyms.

"Okay, shift your balance onto your right leg," I told myself. Then I began to draw my left foot forward. As soon as I raised it just a smidge, my balance swung wildly and I gripped the bars with both hands. I reset my feet and tried again. Weight to the right foot, lean forward, lift up the left foot. Think, "I love you." My foot came down heavy about three inches ahead of where it had been. My therapist grinned and congratulated me. People in the rehab room started to notice something happening over at the parallel bars. I smiled internally, but I knew this was only one step, and one step was not walking. Never one to be easy on myself, I had decided that two steps were required for it to be considered walking.

My legs were burning with fatigue, heavy lead exhaustion. I couldn't plant my feet squarely on the floor. My therapist saw my dilemma and again invited me to sit down but I declined. I swung my weight back and forth and caught the next forward motion and brought my right foot even with my left. "I love you."

I had walked. Everyone was looking as I leaned on the bar with my hip and raised one arm triumphantly. There was cheering and clapping. Then I collapsed back into my chair exhausted. "You did it, Michael. You walked!" said my physical therapist. I smiled. It wasn't me, it was Linda. I was only returning her love.

Five months later I did walk up that aisle with my new bride. I did it for Linda. I did it out of love. We have been married twenty-four years now.

My grandparents are ninety-six and have been married seventy-four years; I have coffee and cookies with them every week. Long lives and long marriages are traditions I intend to keep.

~Mike Strand

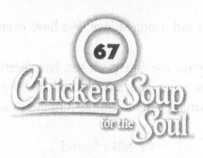

Singing My Way Through Adversity

If music be the food of love, play on.
~William Shakespeare

I first met Shahida Nurullah while recovering from a bad accident where I slipped and fell on treacherous, winter ice in Detroit. I had flown in from sunny Southern California to surprise my hometown friends and my mom. That accident temporarily stopped my life. For six weeks I used a walker; for six more I was on crutches. My jazz singing career was put on hold. Worst of all, I was losing money every day and I was depressed. I had to call and try to save all my upcoming scheduled concerts by sending substitutes. As a self-employed singer who was in perfect health before this accident, I wasn't prepared for illness and I had no health insurance.

One day, concerned friends told me about Shahida Nurullah and suggested I talk to her about my depression. They said Shahida was a woman who had beat the odds and like me, was a successful, working jazz vocalist. That prompted a telephone call and we've been friends ever since. I soon realized that my broken ankle and ultimate bankruptcy were nothing compared to what Shahida Nurullah had gone through.

"I don't really remember, but I'm told I was hit by a car while crossing the street," she told me over the phone.

Shahida's voice was warm, melodic, but tinged with the pain of remembering a traumatic time.

"I awoke in the hospital with no idea what had happened to me. When I first regained my memory, I had problems speaking. I had no idea if I would ever sing again and I said, 'This just won't do! I'm a singer, so I have to be able to speak. I have to be able to sing.'"

"I know you're frustrated right now," she told me empathetically. "Why don't you come over and visit me?"

The next day I went to visit my new friend. I found it so amazing that after her accident she couldn't even speak clearly, because now she was very articulate. Shahida put on a pot of tea and invited me out to her yard. She said she was going to feed the birds. I followed her to a small, lush back yard. She had a beautiful, hand-carved, African cane and she walked proudly, but carefully.

"They expect me to be out here at a certain time," she told me.

I watched as she sprinkled birdseed into her palm, set the big bag of seeds down and then stood motionless in her yard under a lovely shade tree, arms outstretched. A black-capped Chickadee appeared, landed on her open hand, then trustingly fed from her palm. That did it for me. Anyone whom wild animals trusted had to have an open and loving heart. After feeding the birds we settled down on her sunny patio to sip our tea and talk. She continued sharing her miraculous story with me.

"It was a cold, January day in Detroit. I was on my way to my job at Gayle's Chocolates in Royal Oak, an affluent suburb of Detroit. I was humming a song in my head. You know how we singers do it, girl. We're always hearing music in our heads. It was 1989, just two years after I had recorded as part of Geri Allen's Open on All Sides band. Our recording got good reviews. Did you hear it? Do you know Geri? She's a critically acclaimed pianist from Detroit, but now she lives in New York. Anyway, my career seemed to be climbing a golden staircase to success."

Shahida reached underneath her small tea table and pulled out a folded paper, handing it to me. I read the review.

The tour de force "I Sang a Bright Green Tear For All Of Us This Year" *is stunning, featuring the wonderful vocals of Shahida Nurullah, insistent rhythm, haunting refrains from Allen's keyboards, and shifting dynamics that are compelling. www.murfie.com.*

"I was rushing across Van Dyke and Kerchavel Streets to catch my bus," she continued. "They say I was struck by a speeding Cadillac. My injuries were extensive. When I finally awoke from a coma, two and a half weeks later, the doctors told me I had a broken arm, leg, knee, and shoulder and a brain injury that affected my speech and memory. Shocked and frightened, the first thought I had was 'has my voice been affected? Can I still sing?'

"Then I thought about my brother. I became a surrogate parent to him after we lost both our mother and father at a young age. What would happen to him if I didn't heal? I was his protector.

"It took months of rehab and I still have memory issues. I don't limp, but my walk is different and I have to use a cane."

She pointed to an umbrella rack full of artistically designed walking sticks. "I have one for every occasion, even the stage." She laughed, letting soft, red-painted lips spread across her face like bright sunshine.

"But look what I've accomplished. Despite my challenges, I'm working. I've released a solo CD and it's gotten rave reviews. I'm teaching vocals at the University of Windsor and I was nominated for the Kresge Eminent Artist Award in the Performing and Literary Arts. Last year I sang the national anthem at Tiger Stadium and I'm reaching my biggest audience currently, through radio and television ads for Detroit Medical Center. They're celebrating their brand new Neuroscience Unit in the Rehabilitation Institute of Michigan. I'm singing the Four Tops' 'Reach Out, I'll Be There.' I sing it my way; a jazzy way."

I sat there with my crutches on the floor near my chair and my foot wrapped knee-high in a blue boot, blatantly reminding me of my own injury.

"You're blessed." Shahida saw me staring at my leg. "Your ankle will heal and you will sing your way through this, just like I did.

You have the strength of character, the love of your art and the determination to keep going," she affirmed and took a sip of her tea.

"Like me, you have dreams. We have music. Music is healing. It wasn't easy, but the DMC Rehabilitation brought me back with occupational, physical, and speech therapy. They gave me back my voice. They gave me back my life. More than twenty-three years later, I still go there for therapy. Brain injury is no joke! But I believe every experience is a blessing, a lesson of life, and helps us grow stronger and wiser. In a few more weeks, you'll be good as new."

When I left Shahida's house I felt stronger, a whole lot more positive and tremendously encouraged. Six weeks later, I was back in shoes and writing a musical play. Shahida Nurullah became one of my stars and guess what? Like everything else Shahida seems to touch, the play became a critically acclaimed event. We sang our way through it.

~Dee Dee McNeil

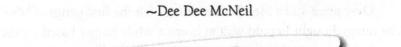

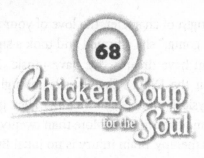

Choosing Emily

A very small degree of hope is sufficient to cause the birth of love.

~Stendahl

I went into labor on a Friday night, December 15, 1989, and my husband Peet was scared. It was nearly a week past my due date and the snow was starting to fall.

Over pizza and a Mel Gibson video, I felt the first pangs of labor. The nurse thought I could wait at home a while longer based on the time between contractions. But the snow started falling harder. Since we lived on a one-lane dirt road, one of the last to be plowed in our rural New Hampshire town, we thought it best to get to the hospital sooner.

As we pulled out of our driveway around midnight, Peet looked at our small antique cape and at the shingled barn, which was built into the gentle slope of a hillside. It looked like a Currier & Ives scene, with our apple orchard trimmed in snow. He choked up a little as he started to talk. I expected him to say something sweet and reassuring. Instead his voice found its deepest register and was serious. "Whatever happens, when we return here, our life will never be the same again," he said.

I knew he was trying to be brave and honor the moment, while at the same time preparing stoically for the worst. What if there were complications with the birth? What if the baby was born with disabilities? What if the child was difficult or sickly?

We'd spent a lot of time during the previous three years playing "what if." Peet's traumatic brain injury in 1986 had left him with cognitive and behavioral issues that hadn't fully resolved. His memory was sometimes spotty. His words did not always come smoothly or quickly. And he had not regained all of his stamina after the one-story fall in our barn, which resulted in emergency brain surgery to remove a subdural hematoma.

We'd learned firsthand how lives could change in an instant. Peet's words made me realize that as I'd gone into labor, he worried about facing another pivotal moment. It was more than the typical worry about something going wrong with the baby's delivery. I knew he was concerned that lingering issues from his brain injury would prevent him from being a good father. Still, we'd decided together to try, more than a year before.

Like most young couples, we'd done everything we could to ensure the arrival of a healthy newborn. We'd checked with doctors to be sure that the anti-seizure medication Peet used after his injury would not impact his fertility or the health of the baby. I'd eaten wholesome foods. I exercised routinely, swimming laps until days before the birth.

Still his "whatever happens" comment echoed in my head as we crawled along on unplowed roads for the half-hour drive to the hospital. We both stared silently at the small path that the headlights carved for us in the whitened night, as if our concentration could get us there more safely. When we made it up the final hill that led to the hospital in Peterborough, we breathed a sigh of relief.

Peet was unable to stay awake while I was in labor during the next several hours. His need to sleep at least ten hours a night simply overwhelmed him. I spent the night going in and out of the whirlpool tub for relief, watching him nap on the chair in our hospital suite.

By mid-morning I was fully dilated and Peet was wide-awake by my side. Minutes from delivery though, things got tense. I was not having the urge to push as I should. Even when guided by the nursing staff to push hard, the baby was not budging. It turned out that one of the baby's arms was extended alongside her head in the birth canal and the umbilical cord was around her neck. The doctor asked for permission to use a vacuum extractor—a sort of suction cup attached to the baby's head to help a doctor pull a baby out while the mother pushes. The first few tries with the vacuum extractor did not work. I knew that the next step might be forceps. I had always heard that forceps were riskier and had a chance of causing brain damage. We couldn't use forceps. The doctor tried the vacuum extractor one more time, yelling "push" with an added sense of urgency.

Emily arrived.

They put her on my chest and she began nursing almost instantly. Her hazel eyes were a kaleidoscope of beauty, intensity and curiosity, as they are today. She was alert and content. Peet and I wept.

Within an hour, Peet went home to get some rest. I watched through the second-story window of my hospital room as he brushed about eight inches of snow off my old red Saab and drove away. Vibrant blue skies contrasted with the blanket of snow, which was literally sparkling in the daylight.

Alone that afternoon, I noticed the shape of Emily's head. It was cone-shaped and a little bruised, which I knew was not uncommon. Still I was concerned. I'd been so happy at her arrival that I'd forgotten to ask the doctor if there could be anything wrong that resulted from her difficult time in the birth canal.

I got up the nerve to ask the doctor about Emily's head, explaining that my husband had suffered a brain injury years before. I needed reassurance that the baby was fine. "Completely normal," he said. "A 9 on the Apgar scale. She's practically perfect."

The next day, a Sunday, we were serenaded in the maternity ward by Boy Scouts singing Christmas carols. We watched a Buffalo Bills football game, our favorite team, and Peet made a spaghetti dinner for us in the little hospital kitchen. We feasted on Ben and Jerry's Cherry Garcia ice cream.

As we left the hospital the following morning, we shared an elevator with two elderly hospital volunteers. Bundled in homemade knit hats and scarves and weighing about a hundred pounds each, the women reminded me of Santa's elves.

"Is this your first baby?" one of them asked, clearly delighted.

Peet and I looked at each other, grinned, and nodded sheepishly. No doubt I was holding the baby protectively at an unnatural angle, afraid I would break her. To the outside world, we were just an average set of newly minted parents. How good it felt to be average.

"There is nothing more special than a Christmas baby," the other woman added before saying goodbye with gentle finger waves.

We drove back home with Emily sleeping peacefully in her new carseat. The roads were clear and dry. As we pulled into the driveway to bring our daughter home, I recalled Peet's words from a few nights before and heard them differently this time. He'd been right. Our life would never be the same again, in the best possible way.

~Tina Rapp

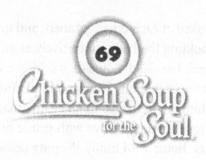

69

A God-Colored Lens

The pessimist sees the difficulty in every opportunity. The optimist sees the opportunity in every difficulty.
~Winston Churchill

My daughter's features resembled those in a Picasso painting—catatonic eyes somewhat askew and a face void of expression save for the slight smile that twitched on only one side. She couldn't talk, couldn't walk and, at the age of eighteen, was wearing a diaper. How could it be possible that my beautiful girl would ever be the same? The reality was that she wouldn't. But by the grace of God and a strong will, she would be better than her pre-traumatic brain injury self.

The car accident that landed Nicole in a coma occurred on December 18, 2003. She spent a week in the ICU and awoke on Christmas morning. My prayers were answered, but God never leaves well enough alone. He often has a better plan. For the next seven weeks, she spent her time in rehab learning everything all over again.

The progress was slow—two steps forward, one step back. Journaling helped me keep a healthy perspective. My honor student daughter struggled with the Tupperware Shape-O Ball—a toy she hadn't played with since she was two. She had memory loss, was unable to identify simple items, and didn't speak coherently for three weeks.

And yet, my spirited, intelligent daughter was alive and well, even if she was unable to communicate. I made the usual ninety-minute commute one morning to the inpatient rehabilitation hospital and arrived in the aftermath of chaos. Nicole's occupational therapist was flushed and flustered.

"Nicole's fine," Veronica said, before I could even ask. "But I'm afraid she escaped."

"Escaped?" I stepped around her and made a beeline for Nicole's room, my heart beating in triple time. There Nicole was, asleep on her bed, curled into a fetal position.

Veronica stepped into the room. "We're taking precautions."

"I don't understand how this could have happened."

"She wheeled her wheelchair to the back door and out she went."

"But you assured me that an alarm would sound if she opened the door."

A smile played over Veronica's lips. "There is a definite positive here. She removed the monitor from her chair."

I glanced at Nicole's wheelchair sitting in the corner of the sterile room. There had been a small monitor strapped to the bottom—which was supposed to sound an alarm if the hospital doors were opened. It was no longer there.

"How is that positive?"

"It took planning," Veronica said. "Don't you see? She's not even talking yet, but she knew the monitor would impede her escape. She figured out how to remove it and then found her way to the back door. It was brilliant."

Brilliant.

Veronica threw her hands up. "We just have to outsmart her."

When Nicole left the hospital the first week of February, she was walking and talking. And talking. And talking. Not much different than before the accident. However, we discovered the real work was just beginning.

Focus was an issue. She couldn't stay with any activity, such as reading or eating; yet if her emotions were involved, she could focus on nothing else. It was like living with Sarah Bernhardt. Friends, who didn't understand that Nicole had lost her filter system and wasn't trying to be insulting, abandoned her, leading to more heartache, drama and confusion.

But we retained our sense of humor.

Dressed and ready to head out for an outpatient therapy appointment, Nicole presented herself to me.

"You look very cute," I told her.

"Yeah." She patted her slacks-clad thighs. "My shirt matches my balls."

I must have misheard her. "Excuse me?"

"My shirt." She plucked at the gauzy top. "It matches my balls." Again, she patted her thighs.

"Pants, sweetheart. You're wearing pants."

Nicole had always wanted to be a writer, and now she struggled with finding simple words. Word-smithing was reduced to elementary vocabulary. Her speech therapist told me that the more intelligent the individual, the harder it was to accept the new "normal." She would be aware of her limitations, and that would be extremely frustrating for her. Eight months of bi-weekly speech therapy appointments gave her the tools to handle the short-term memory loss. However, breezing through college courses, as she had before the accident, was a thing of the past.

A year after her accident, Nicole moved closer to college. The commute was too strenuous. She was taking a few classes and working as a cashier at a gas station grocery store. She called me in tears one afternoon.

"This guy came in," she sobbed. "He was really rude. I was trying to figure out how much change he had coming. I messed up yesterday and just wanted to get it right. He told me I was stupid. 'Why would they hire some imbecile who can't even count?' he said," her voice breaking.

"Oh, Nicole. It's okay." But it wasn't. Tears formed in my own eyes while anger surged through my body.

"No, Mom, it's not okay. I used to be smart."

This was the hardest thing for Nicole—to watch her friends fly through college while she struggled with basic math. To know that she had a plan and a purpose in her life that no longer fit.

But God had a new plan—and it started in the form of a guardian angel. Danny is an intelligent young man who was able to see past Nicole's focus issues, lack of a filtering system and occasional bouts of emotionalism. He encourages her with love and humor to look past what others might deem a disability. She's come to see it not as a disability, but a challenge God has given her.

They have been married for six years now, and at the end of last year they moved to Louisiana when Danny accepted a job transfer. Nicole, who completed her associate's degree a few classes at a time, is now pursuing a bachelor's degree in English. Last summer, she was hired as a library assistant.

"Miss Judy just told me why I was hired," Nicole informed me on the phone a few weeks ago. "She said there were a lot of applicants who were more qualified, but she sensed a special spirit in me."

"I'm not at all surprised."

A memory flitted through my head—Nicole's therapists at the hospital telling me how she was different. "Most of the young people we see are victims of car accidents because they're drinking or doing drugs. They're angry to start with, and the TBI just exacerbates the situation. But Nicole? She's always smiling and saying, 'please' and 'thank you.' What a breath of fresh air she is."

The accident that nearly took my daughter's life gave her the heart and compassion to see people through a different lens—a God-colored lens. She's different—not because she lives with traumatic brain injury, but because she's lived through an experience that has forever changed her.

—Jennifer Sienes

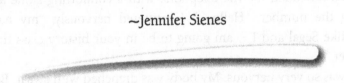

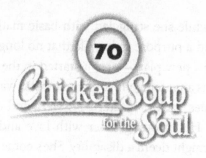

Butch

Our greatest weakness lies in giving up. The most certain way to succeed
is always to try just one more time.
~Thomas A. Edison

I remember it as if it were yesterday, but it occurred so many years ago. Maria, my speech pathologist, was practicing with me for a very important phone call. "All right, say it again," Maria would repeat time after time, trying to help me with my rate, tempo, speed, as well as my nerves.

Months prior to these sessions, few thought I would survive, much less be practicing for this phone call. I had been severely brain-injured in a robbery when one of three thieves shot me in the head. He thought he had eliminated every witness; he was wrong. I had to relearn to do so much: walk, talk, and do so many things that normal people take for granted.

Almost fourteen months since that eventful night, I was practicing for the phone call that I would make to explain my situation to my first teacher in college since the shooting.

Maria handed me the telephone with a comforting smile after dialing the number. "Hello..." I muttered nervously, "my name is... Mike Segal and I... am going to be in your history class this... summer."

I was so very nervous. My body was drenched with sweat. But I slowly went on to explain my situation and the fact that I might need extra time to take exams. I never expected the response I got.

"Come on, Johnny. I know this is a joke."

I broke down sobbing and screaming, "Mister, I wish this was a joke!"

Seeing my reaction, Maria quickly grabbed the phone and sternly said, "This is Maria Dantoni. I am Mike's speech pathologist at Del Oro Institute for Rehabilitation." She quickly repeated what had happened to me and said, "Mike was very proud that he finally might be able to resume his classes. However, he appears to be very upset by what you have just said. What did you say?"

The history teacher was crushed. He thought it was a joke and explained to Maria, "Ma'am, when I was in college a few years ago, my roommates and I used to play practical jokes on each other. We still do. I could have sworn that one of my old roommates, John, was just playing a joke. I am so, so sorry."

I was still sobbing while Maria was listening to his explanation. Many people, I would imagine, would have remained crushed after hearing his response. But I refused to let his comments permanently get me down.

I showed up in room 112 on a warm summer evening to begin my classes with Mr. Butch Johnson as my teacher. It was not simply a question of taking the class; for me, it was a huge hurdle as it would determine whether or not I was cognitively and physically ready to resume my college life, as well as get on with my life in general.

And Butch Johnson was wonderful. He made sure I understood everything in his class. Whatever I needed during the first week of class, he made sure I received it. After one week, we were scheduled to have our first exam. The closer we came to the exam date, the more nervous I became.

Finally, the test day arrived. I was so nervous sitting at my desk before the exam. It had been well over a year since I had taken a college exam. What kind of grade would I make? Would I do okay? I became more and more anxious.

Butch (he had told me that I could call him Butch, rather than Mr. Johnson) handed me the exam first. I looked at it. It consisted of a variety of short answers as well as several multiple-choice questions.

Since I was not sure of the first answer (a fact that did not ease my nerves) I went on to question 2, promising myself to return to the first question before I turned in the exam. I was busy trying to answer the questions when I noticed people turning in their tests. When I finally finished my test, the classroom was empty and all the other students were gone.

Finally, about thirty minutes after the bell had rung, I limped up to his desk to turn in my exam.

The next evening at school, Butch passed out the graded exams. I was so fidgety and tense. I thought, "What if I failed? Maybe it was too early for me to try school." I was full of negative doubts.

Just then, Butch came to my desk, handed me my exam with a smile and said, "Congratulations, Mike."

I looked down at my desktop and saw a red letter "C" written on my test. Before the shooting, I would have been very upset with a "B," much less a "C." But I was smiling from ear to ear with that passing grade. I had done it. I had passed my first exam!

After that first test, I made all "A's" in that history class. But I was most proud of that first "C," as it showed me, as well as so many others, that I was ready to return to the world.

Four years after that first history class, I graduated with honors from the University of Texas at Austin. The moral of this story is not just about an injured teenager returning to college. Rather it is the lesson that everyone should always try to do his best. I've learned firsthand that excelling in life is not vital, but trying is! Sometimes, a "C" can be just as precious as an "A"!

~Michael Jordan Segal, MSW

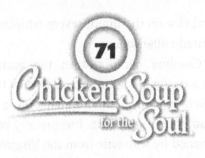

Sometimes
the Little Fish Wins

A person without a sense of humor is like a wagon without springs.
It's jolted by every pebble in the road.
~Henry Ward Beecher

Never lie to your parents. It always comes back to bite you in the butt, especially the big ones (the lies, not the butts.) Many years ago, I told my parents I was going on vacation to Wisconsin with a girlfriend. In truth, I was driving alone from our family home in Chicago to a North Carolina military base to visit a boyfriend (whom they didn't like) who was stationed there. Had I known I'd end up in a head-on car crash on my way home, almost losing my life, I'd have gone to Wisconsin!

On an icy bridge, my lightweight car ricocheted off another vehicle. It jumped the guardrail and slid down a forty-foot snow-slicked embankment, coming to rest at the bottom on railroad tracks. I broke the front seatback and flew like a human rocket, smashing the right rear door open with my head. This happened in the days before seatbelt laws. The engine ended up in the front seat where I would have been had I been seatbelted.

I lay near death several yards away from where I had been launched, and my brand-new car was totaled just a couple of weeks after I'd made the last payment on it (surely punishment for lying).

I sustained a blood clot on the brain, severe whiplash, several lacerations, and a fractured collarbone.

The North Carolina clinic nearest the accident site wasn't equipped to treat a traumatic brain injury, so they transferred me by funeral hearse (their version of an ambulance) to a large hospital in Virginia, better equipped to treat me. Imagine my parents' confusion after being telephoned by someone from the Virginia hospital telling them I'd been in an accident in North Carolina and that I needed emergency brain surgery to save me.

They were urged to make their flight arrangements immediately and wait for the neurosurgeon to call back. Several hours passed, and in the middle of the night, the doctor called, advising my folks to get there quickly while he tried to keep me alive.

Early the next morning, they took three connecting flights, arriving in Roanoke, Virginia, late in the afternoon. The young girl at the hospital information desk said in her sweetest Southern drawl, "Oh, y'all are the parents of the deceased?"

My parents gasped, "What?"

Realizing her mistake, the poor girl stammered, "Oh, I'm sorry! I meant the patient in a coma," and then quickly gave them my room number.

My mother and dad rushed to my room and froze in the doorway. They didn't recognize me because my shaved head was cocooned in a turban-like surgical bandage, and my face and body had turned black from bruising.

I remained in a coma for ten days and, even so, tried repeatedly to scratch out my IV and then claw the nurse attempting to reinsert it. When I finally regained consciousness, I would find that my fingernails had been clipped short and splints strapped beneath my arms to prevent further injury to me or my nurses. I also discovered I had double vision, partial paralysis on one side, no memory at all of having the accident, and no car.

The first time I tried to walk on my own, my doctor held his arms out to me. But I was more concerned about keeping my hospital gown closed in back than I was about walking to him. Those hospital gowns don't leave much to the imagination. I suppose that's where they got the term "ICU."

Weeks later, when I was discharged, we flew home to Chicago. We boarded the aircraft and made our way down the aisle to our seats in the last row. The seatbacks wouldn't recline, and as soon as we settled in, I knew I wouldn't be able to sit ramrod straight throughout the long flight ahead. The flight attendant agreed to move us, but we had to hurry because takeoff was imminent. Without thinking, I quickly stood up, forgetting the overhead compartment was just inches above my head.

I hit the hard ceiling with such force that the pain doubled me in half over the seatback in front of me. I began crying, the wig covering my bald head was askew, and my gauze eye bandage for my double vision became soaked with tears. I thought the flight attendant would faint as well. After all the drama subsided, our seats were changed.

Once home, I needed several months of medical follow-ups as I healed. At one appointment, I sat in the crowded waiting room until it was my turn to be seen. After examining me, the doctor decided to administer a cortisone injection in the back of my neck to ease the lingering pain from the whiplash injury. I screamed the entire time it took him to give me the shot, once again soaking my eye bandage with tears. When I left the examining room, there wasn't a soul there. Who knew I could yell loud enough to clear an entire waiting room?

In the weeks that followed, I regained my strength, and life returned to normal. Special eyeglass lenses finally controlled my double vision, which disappeared entirely after about six months. I've never fully recovered my memory, and I'm also at that age now where I've entered the "Wonder Years"—I wonder what I'm going to forget next! But maintaining a positive outlook (plus several datebooks and calendars) has helped me deal with the effects of the traumatic brain injury and get on with life. I guess you can say for me "TBI" means "To Be Inspired."

Back at work, I had continuing difficulty with my memory, a residual effect of the traumatic brain injury. What other people took for granted—learning new assignments or remembering everyday routines—slipped quickly from my recall. My supervisor was very understanding, though. When he found I hadn't completed certain tasks, he tactfully suggested I keep a notebook. I could use it to add entries to help remember the things I had to accomplish during the workday. All was well and good—that is, until I forgot where I put the notebook!

Some people grow plants in an office, but I kept a fishbowl of guppies, one of whom was very pregnant. I monitored her advancement daily, and prepared a smaller fishbowl beside the larger one in anticipation of the delivery day. I knew to retrieve the guppies as they were born because I'd read that the fish ate their young soon after delivering.

As my supervisor conducted our weekly staff meeting, I sat recording the meeting notes when mama began cranking out the newborn fishies. It's not that I wasn't expecting it. I just forgot to look up from my notetaking. By the time I remembered, it was too late. I jumped up from my chair and raced toward the fishbowl just as she gulped down all but one. That experience taught me a valuable lesson: Sometimes you're the big fish and sometimes you're the bait. It's all about endurance in life, and sometimes you have to work hard and swim like mad just to survive.

~Annette Langer

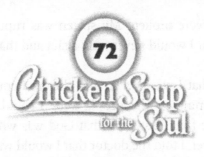

My Ray of Sunshine

Being deeply loved by someone gives you strength.
Loving someone deeply gives you courage.
~Lao Tzu

Life is as good as you make it. I made the most of my time and I loved my life, fitting work, school, homework, and fun with my family and friends into my busy schedule. I was an outgoing, energetic, fun-loving twenty-something, with an optimistic attitude and strong faith. I valued my relationships and worked hard at achieving my goals.

I was living with a close friend while working at a few jobs to put myself through university and become an elementary school teacher. In my last semester, life turned upside down. It was a clear morning on September 25th in 2009. I was working as a traffic controller, wearing my high-visibility gear. As I was holding up my stop sign, I was hit by an SUV at approximately eighty kilometers per hour. I am 5'0" tall and weighed 120 pounds. I flew across the street, out of my steel-toe boots, and landed in front of my coworker.

I was in critical condition. I am told that I technically died but was revived while being airlifted to the hospital. I was admitted to the intensive care unit where I was in an induced coma for six days. After several surgeries, the medical reports indicated that I had bilateral carotid artery dissection and severe brain damage to my frontal lobe, occipital lobe and hypothalamus. In addition, my pelvis was shattered, all of my ribs were cracked, and my sternum, sacrum, cheek, nose, and arm were broken. My spleen was ruptured. The doctor informed me that I would never walk again and that I had retrograde amnesia.

I thought that I was in a strange dream. I couldn't understand what was happening or who people were. I could barely move and only knew basic facts. But I felt that God was with me and would help me to recover. I told the doctor that I would walk down the aisle at my wedding someday.

During my recovery at the hospital, I had many visitors. I was informed that one was my boyfriend, so I assumed that it was the guy who I was most attracted to. I was told the name of my boyfriend, so I called the best-looking one by that name… but I was mistaken. Ray was not my boyfriend, but I thought he was perfection! I zealously declared my love for Ray to all of my visitors. My friends told me that I was just confused, but I was certain that he was the one I wanted. This ended the relationship with my unknown boyfriend. Fortunately, Ray drove an hour to visit me every day.

I had only met Ray ten days before the accident, yet it seemed like he was the only person that I could remember. I tried telling him some events that I thought I remembered, but he corrected me. Somehow that caused my brain to switch back into reality. The realization that I hadn't been dreaming had left me extremely confused, but even more surprised that Ray was real! He showed love, patience, kindness, thoughtfulness, and every other virtue that I admired. I recognized how selfless it was for him to support and encourage me, while constantly trying to make me happy.

My memory didn't last longer than the present moments that I was experiencing, so Ray constantly tried to make sure that I felt special. He'd bring me a rose and a slushy drink daily, he'd give me compliments, and he'd take me to get my hair done professionally. Whenever he could, he'd also lie by my side to comfort me. He made me feel unconditionally loved!

Aside from Ray, my life was very difficult. I had lost all of my independence. For a long time, I required help to be fed, bathed, moved, dressed, and even taken to the toilet. I couldn't sleep. I could only lie down or sit in my wheelchair. I had also lost my sense of smell and taste, so I always ate until I was full. This resulted in weight gain. I was very depressed about that. Ray just said there was just more of me to love.

I was slow to process information and my vocabulary was very simple, I couldn't follow people's conversations and I lost my creativity. I also couldn't grasp the concept of time and frequently repeated myself without knowing it. I always felt stupid and confused. Without visual memory, I couldn't distinguish fruits, vegetables, meats, animals, or even people that I should have known. I also often made people feel uncomfortable in conversations by blurting out comments that I didn't know were inappropriate; I didn't have a filter. I'd even interrupt speakers because I couldn't hold onto a thought. Ray noticed my struggles and was aware that I could only retain information with focus and repetition, so he encouraged me to ask questions, he repeated answers, and he summarized previous conversations for me. I had so much to relearn.

Although everything was wonderful with Ray, I yearned for the strong friendships that I had before the accident. I needed to expand my social horizons. I had a hard time paying attention, but I tried my best to focus, listen, and not speak until my turn. When I'd talk, I'd ask basic questions. Each night, I tried to review the day, repeating as much "new" information as I could. I found that the amount of information I was able to remember was increasing daily. I spent all of my time learning. I frequently studied a thesaurus to increase my vocabulary, and Ray regularly played games with me to improve my mental faculty. My brain injury no longer seemed obvious to others.

On the other hand, my physical disabilities continued to limit my independence, so I worked very hard with a kinesiologist to strengthen my muscles and improve my range of motion. I had to push through the pain to stand and take my first step while using a walker. I eventually progressed to a cane. Now, I am proud to say that I don't need any assistance with my walking! I knew what I wanted to do, and I have exceeded all expectations. In May of 2011, Ray and

I blissfully walked down the aisle and now we are expecting our first child!

Through my constant pain and distress, I am still the same girl that I was. Being disabled is tough, and people can't see my cognitive struggles. But with prayer, appreciation, and effort, I will keep moving forward. It is unnecessary to focus on the pain; I focus on positive distractions. I am determined to enjoy my life with my best friend. It's been a challenge in so many ways, but I am grateful that my Ray of sunshine carried me through the storm!

~Jennifer Wiche

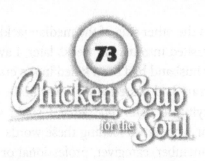

New Life in New York City

The essence of all beautiful art, all great art, is gratitude.
~Friedrich Nietzsche

A-Rod, in his fifth season in the Bronx, was on deck to face the Angels. The crowd, at this point still enamored with their two-time MVP, erupted in a rousing ovation. But it wasn't long before Rodriguez showed signs of fatigue. Yup, he was struggling. To make matters worse, Andy Pettitte was pitching wild and couldn't seem to keep anyone off base. The Yankees had won the previous eight games in a row, and this was one of the last ever to be played in the iconic old Yankee Stadium. The energy and tension were palpable among the fans.

Rich and I were on a newlywed high and no loss could dampen the joy we felt as we huddled together in the stands, sharing plans for a future nursery in our new home and reviewing a to-do list for our dog, Moses. What a summer this would be! At thirty years old, I was already a VP and rising star at a top New York City public relations firm and I was excited about a trip I'd be taking for a client the very next day. Rich, an aspiring singer/songwriter, softly sang one of his new melodies into my ear. It was a night to remember.

Or so I imagine. I have no real memory of that evening or of many of the days and nights that came before and after it.

I am told that Rich and I were at that game. The date was July 31, 2008. The final score was the Los Angeles Angels 12, the New York Yankees 6. It was a devastating loss. As we were driving home, an 18-wheeler on the other side of the median jackknifed over a concrete wall and crashed into us. Six weeks later, I awoke in a strange hospital bed. My husband had been killed in the crash. Our one-year wedding anniversary had passed while I was in the coma.

I've been trying to determine what I could share that would be meaningful for whoever is reading these words. Are you a fellow survivor, family member, caregiver, professional or someone who is facing some other kind of adversity? Are you someone who is looking for a reason to keep moving forward? Since sustaining the traumatic brain injury, I've met some incredible people, perhaps like you, whose stories of strength, resilience and survival have given me both a reason to keep moving forward and a purpose.

I had to make physical and psychological adjustments to the injury, including dealing with cognitive issues and community reintegration. The physical adjustments were enormous. On the day my mother arrived at the hospital, a doctor told her that I had severe injuries to every part of my brain and that I would never walk or talk again. For six weeks, I was strapped to a rotating bed in order to protect a fractured vertebra in my neck. I wore what is called a halo, which is a metal brace screwed into the skull to keep the bones in the cervical spine stable. At one point, it became infected. Believe me, there was nothing angelic about that halo! Just before being discharged, I finally took my first steps into my dad's arms.

As for community reintegration, I reached out to people who had been part of my life before the accident, including my high school prom date, my first intern, business partners, neighbors, colleagues and editors with whom I had worked. Unfamiliar but apparently dear friends visited me in the hospital and sent me cards and flowers. I made it a point to reconnect weekly with a person from the past. I asked each one to tell me who I was. The person they described is whom I now refer to as Angela 1.

The fact is, Angela 1 died after that fateful Yankee game. On the same night, Angela 2 was born. Angela 1 and Angela 2 are very different people.

Angela 1 was a young executive, a new bride and a proud owner of her first home with her first true love. She was unaware that life can change dramatically in an instant. She had memories, a clear history and believed she had a clear future.

Let me introduce Angela 2, who began as a depressed, medicated young widow, without a career, home or independence. As of this writing, Angela 2 still gets lost frequently, sleeps a lot and moves slowly. But she is a rock star who has recovered and grown beyond anyone's expectations, including her own.

Once I was able to embrace these two selves, I stopped trying to wear the shoes of Angela 1. They simply don't fit anymore. Instead, I wholly love and inhabit Angela 2.

I am a big believer in expressing gratitude whenever possible. I'm confident that my life before the accident was filled with as many blessings as it is today. It's just that Angela 2 is more focused and aware of them now. And I no longer have the dubious luxury of sweating the small stuff. After surviving the enormity of what happened, everything else pales in comparison.

Being on a disability schedule has provided me with an opportunity to grow in ways that Angela 1 would never have had the time to explore. For example, I am able to take classes at a spiritual center where I've strengthened my spiritual muscles. I've learned the powerful tool of meditation. As a result, I have successfully navigated my way through anxious moments and situations by quieting the thoughts, stilling the body and relaxing the mind.

I have also learned that by concentrating on the blessings, more blessings come, and that expressing gratitude attracts more reasons to feel grateful.

After the car crash, gifts from across the country poured into my hospital room, and later, to the rehabilitation center where I did my outpatient therapy. At the time, I experienced a mounting anxiety about keeping up with writing all the thank-you notes as Angela 1 would have. Only later did I finally recognize that I was the recipient of an outpouring of love. Only then did I allow myself to truly receive the blessing and experience the grace of genuine connection.

Angela 2 is happy, present and determined to keep moving forward.

~Angela Leigh Tucker

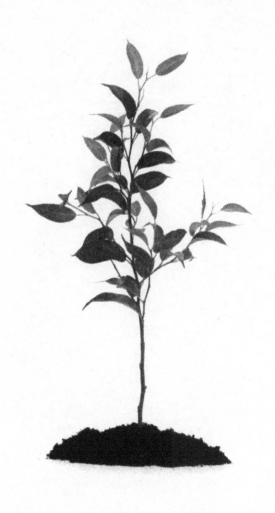

Chapter
8

Recovering *from* Traumatic Brain Injuries

Coping Strategies that Work

Chapter

8

Recovering
from Traumatic
Brain Injuries

Coping Strategies
that Work

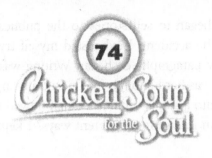
Survive, Revive, Thrive

Take the first step in faith. You don't have to see the whole staircase,
just take the first step.
~Martin Luther King, Jr.

I've driven on icy Ohio roads since I was sixteen. I could always pull myself out of fishtails or push myself out of ditches until December 23rd six years ago. I spun off the road and rolled twice. I woke up to broken glass in my beard, a cold breeze where my driver's side window used to be, and a truck driver trudging toward me through the snow, asking if I was okay.

I was lucky. I was alive. My wife wasn't with me in the car. And though my airbag didn't deploy, my only injuries were a bruise from the seatbelt strap, and what we thought at the time was a simple concussion when my skull shattered the window. No loss of motor skills. No personality changes. Just a concussion.

I vaguely remember a doctor saying it would be a few days before my ability to focus would return to normal. When I was still having trouble weeks later, another doctor told us: "Well, yes, it could be days. Or it could be weeks."

Later: "Could be weeks, could be months."

Then: "Could be months, could be years."

And it was also possible that this would be my life from now on.

I was constantly frustrated. I felt like I was a burden. I was a writer. That was my identity. And years of working at it were finally paying off as I began to sell stories to the publications I'd grown up with. After the accident, I exhausted myself trying to read and retain just a few paragraphs each day. Writing was worse. Subject-verb agreement was hard enough to concentrate on, but assembling multiple ideas into a single sentence which flowed between the previous and next in interesting, coherent ways? I kept at it, but it felt hopeless.

Appropriately, most of the resources out there are for more severe brain injuries. A concussion taking more than five years to go away is more of a strange limbo in which you don't need as much help, but the help you do need is harder to find. How do you ask for help when you don't know what's wrong? And here my luck continued....

A few weeks before my accident, I'd begun writing a brain-related science fiction story, and while perusing my library's neuroscience shelves for research material, I saw a book called *Brainlash*. I liked the title, but it had little to do with my specific topic, so I put it back and forgot about it.

Six months later, I was determined to return to work on that story, no matter how many months or years it would take me to finish. Back at those library shelves, I thought for the second time, "Oh, that's an interesting title." I picked up that same copy of that same book again and looked at the cover. The full title? *Brainlash: Maximize Your Recovery from Mild Brain Injury*. My story research could wait.

Starting with that book, I've learned that I have post-concussion syndrome or an mTBI (mild traumatic brain injury). I've learned about neuropsychiatry and other therapies. Neuro-feedback was helpful in my case. ADHD drugs... not so much. Medicinal levels of caffeine were fantastic in the short term, devastating in the long term. I've optimized my diet with brain-friendly essential fatty acids. I've figured out ways within my limitations to be socially, physically, and mentally active, giving me three chances at neuroplasticity.

I've learned that I'm slowed, but not stopped. It's been gradual, but I'm now able to read entire chapters of novels in one sitting, and have sold stories I've written partially or even entirely post-injury.

Energy management has become more important to me than

time management. I'll look up restaurant menus ahead of time, so I don't tire myself trying to read in front of my friends (or feel embarrassed because I didn't finish looking at the appetizers by the time they're all paying the check). I've learned to be ready with phrases like "I might be fading," which can take some social sting out of asking everyone to please leave me alone because I've got nothing left to offer today.

I've learned to compensate for my weaknesses. Even as I learned to read properly again, I also listen to spoken word audio. It's more passive an activity than reading something on the page, but it is fulfilling. As a scripter of comic books, I now rely more on my illustrator's attention to detail than I do my own. And last year, a story I wrote won an Eagle Award, the longest running of the major comic book industry's honors. My collaborator and I are no less happy for sharing the credit.

Even six years out, there can be weeks of lucidity followed by longer stretches of feeling as bad as I did in those first few months. But by giving each day a score from 1 to 10, and tracking those numbers on a spreadsheet, I can see a moving average of the previous sixty days and see that number improving when the ups and downs day to day make it hard to feel that I'm getting better.

I've learned that everyone has days when they don't feel they measure up. Forgetting where I put my keys was a problem before my accident, too. Everyone's brains disappoint them now and then. I can do anything I set my imperfect but still viable mind to, if I break tasks down into subtasks small enough that they don't overwhelm me.

I tend to speak more rapidly since my bump on the head, and I've realized it's because I lack confidence in the value of what I'm saying. I don't want to waste anyone's time with my brain's meager offerings, so I try to get it over with quickly. I'm working on that.

An author friend told me about this book and its call for essays. I'd met her in Hollywood earlier this year, where she took the grand prize in an international short story competition in which I was a third place winner. By her prose or by social interaction, I wouldn't have known she was dyslexic if she hadn't mentioned it. I'm sure the same is true for me and my hurdle.

Today, I apologize less often for being slow. I used to explain that I'm recovering from a head bump in order to blunt the unpleasantness of my quirks. As it turns out, my bringing it up would often provide the first hint of awkwardness in a conversation. Oops.

Immediately after the accident, my focus was on survival. Over months and then years, I was lucky enough to move beyond that, on to how best to revive my former abilities.

Now, though I may never regain everything I've lost, I don't spend all my time fighting for it anymore either.

I want to thrive. And I'm lucky to be able to want that.

~Lex Wilson

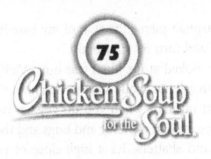

75

Yoga Love

Yoga teaches us to cure what need not be endured
and endure what cannot be cured.
~B.K.S. Iyengar

"Janna Marie?" I heard my dad's footsteps shift the floorboards. I looked at the clock—6:32 a.m. I rolled over into the freshly laundered pillows that my mother always stacked on my bed. Four hours was no longer enough sleep. I had to work for my thoughts, cracking them open like pistachios.

"It's your birthday today," he said, now standing in my doorway.

Oh no. Thirty! Right here. Right now. Today.

My heart squeezed tight. Something like camel pose would help this. One long, languid heart-opener, bearing it all to the Pennsylvania sun, would nip this anxiety.

"Are you going to get up and teach us yoga?"

"Dad, it's not seven yet." I lifted myself up to sit straight. "We said seven."

"We'll wait for you in the driveway," he said, heading back down the stairs.

I slipped into leggings and a tank top and padded down to the kitchen to grab my aviators and a cup of steaming black coffee. I found my students (my parents and our family friend Vicky) standing obediently in Mountain Pose at the top of their new mats, which sat atop old towels to keep the driveway from scuffing them.

"Um… good morning." I walked in front of them, feeling every contour of the asphalt pierce the skin of my bare feet. "Come to the top of your mat and turn off your brain."

My mother looked at me like I was nuts. Vicky picked up a cat and proceeded to ask me about what to do about the cats. There are barn cats that sit on mats when you do yoga at my parents' house. And birds and our golden retriever and bugs and the occasional pine-cone that falls and shatters. It's a high dose of pratyahara—with-drawing the senses—with nature. My dad stepped forward and puts his palms together at his heart.

Driveway yoga was his idea. He had taken to yoga with an enthu-siasm I thought had long since died in him. Perhaps it's a product of his Beatles Maharishi days, or maybe it's because it's the only thing that doesn't overtax his injured brain.

Everything in his life requires a prompt, a list, a plea. We are constantly reminding him to be more patient, more compassionate, more aware, less compulsive, less demanding, less angry—forever finding ways to lessen the cognitive, emotional and behavioral defi-cits that come with a severe frontal lobe traumatic brain injury. It's a seventeen-year oscillation between failure and semi-success when it comes to finding pieces of Old John.

But yoga works. We started a few years ago, when with a certifi-cation under my belt—proof that I knew what the heck I was doing repositioning a brain-injured man who moved like cement—the right parties gave me permission to teach my father yoga.

"Mom, just let me try it with him," I had said. "I really think he'll gain a lot from it, a lot of things that he needs to work on: self-discipline, his patience, his motivation, his identity, his purpose. Oh, and he'll probably lose weight." She said okay. She really wanted him to lose weight, if nothing else.

"Are you ready for this?" I had asked. It was our first time, and my voice sounded too much like my mother's.

He sat down on the steps, waiting as I pondered how it would be most feasible to do yoga in my parents' hallway. He said nothing, just sat and watched me choose a spot for the mat and stomp it flat.

"Okay, come to the top of your mat." He stood up, the hardwood floor creaking under his 205 pounds. I watched his feet shuffle tiny steps toward his mat. He didn't wear bare feet well, not like he used to. His feet were old, stiff, and he moved them as if they were two bricks attached to the bottom of his legs rather than feet. He stood on his mat, facing his fish tank.

"Not like that." I put my hands on his shoulders, turned him and tapped the top of the mat with my toes, perfectly manicured with red polish. "Like this. Face forward, the front steps. This is the top of your mat."

"Okay," he said.

"Now, bring your hands like this—prayer position." I brought my hands together in front of my chest, the flesh of my palms, fingers and wrists perfectly flush. "In front of your heart."

"Okay."

He sounded so obedient, but he looked like the leaning tower of Pisa, tilted, crumbling, old.

His hands met mismatched in front of his chest, fingers like tangled brambles, growing from knotted and knobby knuckles. I was reminded of the various post-accident incidents involving mowers and band saws.

His left foot jutted out to one side. His hip sank down on the right. He had no butt, and the straighter he tried to stand the bigger his belly grew. His thin arms looked like raw chicken wings. I couldn't find his shoulders. I palmed the flesh around where the collarbone and scapula met and concluded that the muscle was gone. Wrinkles under his chin piled in folds. He held his head back, too far back, too rigid.

"Dad, okay. This is called Ta-da-san-a."

He fought his speech until he could say the word right.

I worked from his feet to the crown of his head, demonstrating the way each body part should face and feel. Slowly, deliberately. I moved each stiff appendage and shifted his torso. His body resisted. It was like trying to work with old, hardened clay.

As we talked about weight and balance, tension and muscles, I thought about the last time I had felt the movement in my father's body. Years, at least. A decade? My eyes welled up. I felt ashamed of the daughter I'd become. He was an extremely loving and affectionate person. And he was a really good hugger. He filled my childhood with hugs. The hugs didn't happen anymore, and that was my fault. It felt funny to hug him, my efforts half-hearted, wrapping one arm around his shoulder kissing him on the cheek, like I was saying goodbye to someone on a New York City sidewalk.

Yoga would be a new kind of affection I could share with him, something good for us both. He tried each pose I chose. He let me help him and move him when he didn't understand. He even asked questions. Two full hours, taxing on both his body and his mind. Taxing on mine, too. But we had yoga. Something we could share. Something that was trying, cumbersome, unfamiliar, and, in time, utterly satisfying.

The sleep had worn off my voice by the time I was counting breaths in Warrior Two, as I guided my driveway yogis. Vicky was strong. My mother was flexible. My father had more concentration, patience, and ease than the two of them put together. My father had found his stride.

For months, my father struggled through basic poses. Yet he kept at it, unearthing hints of identity, motivation, and purpose through his practice. "There is nothing else like yoga," he will tell you. "Nothing else gets the mind and the body to connect like that." He comes to his mat. He moves. He breathes. He feels. He thinks.

He is my greatest gift as a teacher.

~Janna M. Leyde

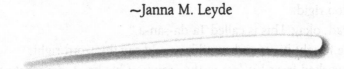

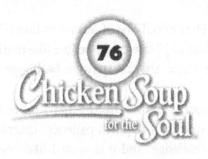

76

Fantastic Frank

Ability is what you're capable of doing. Motivation determines what you do.
Attitude determines how well you do it.
~Lou Holtz

I walked Fantastic Frank to my front door, and resisted the urge to help him put on his jacket and shoes. Whenever he does something that requires coordination, it always looks to me like he is about to fall over, but he never does. We smiled, and he said "Michele, why did we get together today?" I was dumbstruck. "Frank, we just spent four hours together. You really don't remember what we worked on?"

His nervous laugh and flushed cheeks said it all. For the thousandth time I told myself "You must remember he has a traumatic brain injury. Where's your compassion?" To spare him from having to answer, I reminded him that we just had a detailed strategy session about his passion to "Inspire Millions." We reviewed his TV appearances, speaking engagements, website, videos, radio shows, testimonials, and book projects. We looked back at his breakthroughs from the past year, and looked forward to what he wants to accomplish next.

Oh, yes. Now he remembered. He just needed a little nudge and it all came back. All smiles again. "Michele, I am so blessed to work with you. I love you." That always kills me. I get impatient with him, and he says something nice back. I held my son up to say goodbye to Fantastic Frank, closed the door, and sat down.

I was upset. How could I be of service to him if he didn't remember what we worked on? How could he live like that? What kept him going, week after week, always trying to be bigger and reach more people?

Helping Fantastic Frank requires that I move beyond my frustration about his quirks. It requires patience, listening carefully, and love. This is my challenge, and it is what I like best about working with him. It helps me grow as a person.

How can I put myself in his shoes, to better understand him? What is it like having a traumatic brain injury? Sometimes I run upstairs to get something, and in the five or ten seconds it takes to get to the top of the steps, I've forgotten what it was. Is it like that, which is merely annoying, but magnified to every area of your life, all day long, each and every day?

I remember when I met Fantastic Frank for the first time. I was standing in a very long, very slow, line at the department of motor vehicles. Most people looked rather dull, gray, bored, or annoyed. My smiles of happy expectant motherhood met blank faces, and I took to considering baby names while shifting my weight from one foot to the next.

Behind me, standing in the wrong line at the wrong office location, was a gentleman about twenty years my senior, one of the only bright, cheerful faces in the place. He got my attention and introduced himself as "Fantastic Frank." He said he was a motivational speaker, and wanted to talk to me because he was "attracted to my energy."

My curiosity was piqued. What did he say to people to motivate them? I told him that I was an engineer and he said, "So am I!" I said my degree was in chemical engineering and he said, "So is mine!" I said I went to Clarkson University and he said, "So did I!" This was starting to sound suspicious. If his aide hadn't been by his side, validating his story with "yes" nods, I might have turned back around.

We exchanged business cards, and that evening I checked out his website, which verified his story, and put my mind at ease that he was authentic. I called up Fantastic Frank to get together for a networking meeting. Why not? He was a lot more fun to talk to than most people I was meeting in my career search. I had no expectation that this would lead to anything work-wise; I just thought he was interesting.

Like everyone else, I used the back entrance of Fantastic Frank's Tudor style house. The door immediately opened to a few stairs, which put me face to face with a large black dog eagerly greeting me from the kitchen, at the top step. A tour quickly revealed Frank's love of Jack Kirby comic art, with framed pieces and collectible toys displayed throughout the house.

When he mentioned a project he was stuck on, which required transcribing, I blurted out, "I can help with that!"

"I'll even pay you!" he said.

"Even better!" I replied. That's how our work together began: a six-week assignment that became years of one project after the next.

Fantastic Frank is highly intelligent, so sometimes I forget that he has a traumatic brain injury. One of the ways it shows up is that he has a challenge compartmentalizing things. He often makes a voice recording of his ideas for articles, blogs, books, and speeches. Even though he knows the material because he spoke it, it is very challenging for him to edit the content by himself.

Like anyone's brainstorming session, the transcripts are full of incomplete thoughts; they jump from topic to topic, don't have a logical sequence, and repeat content. Fantastic Frank's challenge, having a TBI, is that when he reviews a transcript, the way it jumps around sounds good to him; that's how his brain functions. He's unable to compartmentalize information, and he knows this. With this awareness, he seeks out people with the right skills to compensate for whatever he feels is his weakness.

Another project was to attend his phone-coaching sessions and assist him in completing the assignments, which could be anything from setting up a website to preparing a speech. The problem that Fantastic Frank would run into is that, because of his TBI, he would often get off a coaching call and forget what he was supposed to do or how to go about it. He's been to many high-level workshops all over the country, and it is always a challenge for him, when he returns from a trip, to remember what he learned and put it into action.

Even though he had a highly skilled mentor, and even though he is a highly intelligent and motivated student, they were both disappointed at his lack of progress in achieving his goals. This is where I came in and now, with a team, Fantastic Frank is able to make exponential progress. He even branded me "Marvelous Michele", and it stuck.

Since then, Fantastic Frank has appeared, in his superhero suit, on television sets across the country, inspiring all who see him. If he can, why can't you?

~Michele Camacho

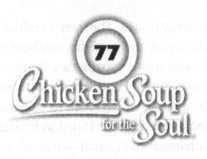

Injury at an Early Age

Once you make a decision, the universe conspires to make it happen.
~Ralph Waldo Emerson

t was 1965 and I was eleven years old. My sixteen-year-old sister was driving, crossing I-35 just north of Liberty, Missouri when the other car T-boned us at an estimated 100 miles per hour. My memories of the following year returned in bits and pieces during my recovery. Almost fifty years later, they are still vivid.

This was before paramedics and ambulances, when funeral homes would often transport the injured. I remember the funeral home attendant—his name was Bud—talking to me as he wrapped me in a blanket and lifted me onto a cot. Bud lifted the cot into the station wagon and sat beside me as we rode to the hospital. I remember a young nurse making a terrible face saying, "Her head is split open." Then she turned and walked away. I remember seeing an operating room with doctors and nurses moving around; there were metal shelves with cloth bundles and instruments. I saw this as if I were sitting on the bright lights hanging from the ceiling. The next thing I remember is my mother helping me count the days before I could leave the hospital. There were thirty-one days marked on the calendar clutched in my hands on the ride home. Later I realized I had been in the hospital for four months. Where did the other 90 days go? Whenever I had questions my entire family would quickly change the subject.

Thankfully I was young enough that the internal injuries and broken bones eventually healed. The three hundred stitches from my right eyebrow to the top of my head left a scar but I could easily cover it with my hair. Sealed inside a body cast for the next six months, I had to relearn how to write and then how to walk. I was voted the "fastest kid on a stick" in reference to using wooden crutches. Personal interactions were difficult. I tried to fit back in with my old crowd but it never happened. I turned to reading or any activity that would keep me in my own little world.

Since then I have spent my time with a very small circle of friends. I still have trouble with large groups. Shopping at our local superstore turns my stomach as I walk through those big doors. I force myself to hold my head up high and look at the faces of people around me. And the knowledge returns that everyone is just as human and sometimes just as frightened as I am. I was never labeled slow or felt any deficit of intelligence; but I lacked ambition. It was the physical limitations I fought, never once considering the possibility of brain injury.

At age fifteen I ran away from home; the year was 1969. The friends I found were heavy into taking acid and drinking alcohol. It took one time trying the mind-bending drug and one time getting drunk to know that they were not for me. I did not like the loss of control over my thoughts and actions. I settled down to smoking pot to fit in. I blame teenage rebellion and enjoying the effects of marijuana for my lack of desire for an education.

My physical limitations qualified me to be tested for financial assistance in finally seeking an education. I passed my GED and completed an associate's degree. I've had a happy and productive professional life.

Fifteen years ago I was diagnosed with a brain tumor. At the time, I was working as a nurse. I was responsible for others' health and wellbeing. I monitored and administered medications and treatments. I felt competent, my superiors agreed and I loved my job. I also understood suffering and being scared to death. I felt qualified to be in the position I held.

I had the tumor removed. It was located directly over the same area as my childhood injury. The doctors could not say if the two were related. During recovery I found myself standing in the shower, unable to decide which faucet was hot and which was cold. I could not remember if the blue bottle was shampoo or body wash. When I reached for the phone, I couldn't remember my mother's phone number. At work I could not remember how to spell the simplest of words.

I could not continue to work in my chosen field if I questioned my abilities, so I had myself tested. The results were above average intelligence, no deficit, no dementia. I went out and bought colored tape, red for the hot faucet, blue for the cold, I bought a huge bottle of body wash and a much smaller shampoo bottle. I taped my mom's phone number under the telephone and at work I started a list of the most common words I used to document patient complaints. These things helped to kick in my memories. Soon I didn't need the reminders. I discovered that when I asked God to return my confidence, He answered me almost immediately. I continued to work as a nurse and in the field of pre-hospital emergency medicine until my recent retirement.

Am I just the luckiest person in the world, to have survived brain injury twice? Medical science knows less about the brain than any other organ in the body.

I have joy and laughter, good friends and family, and the desire to overcome any obstacle. I take each challenge piece by piece, and I inch my way along until I get it right. Yes, baby steps. That's how I learned to walk and write again at age eleven and it is how I accomplish things today. Do I believe in complete and total recovery from a brain injury against all odds? Absolutely, without question or doubt.

~Cheryl Richards

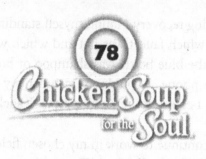

78

The Red Cow House

Inspiration exists, but it has to find us working.
~Pablo Picasso

My dad and I had walked halfway around the empty lake enjoying the silence. I loved the way the sun reflected off the water as dusk approached. My black Lab, Brady, was wading and ducking his head under the water, splashing as he chased fish or perhaps just his own shadow.

At the lake, I could watch the ducks and birds, feel the gentle breeze, and just let myself be. Since the car crash, relaxing activities had been hard to enjoy. Numerous previous concussions had caused only headaches, but this concussion was a doozy.

Post-concussion syndrome was my doctor's diagnosis. As a result, everything became a challenge. Every day, a friend, my mom, or my dad would help me with basic skills and coach me through therapy.

That afternoon, my mother and I had been sitting at the table and she suggested I clean the kitchen. I looked at the kitchen and figured out what needed to be done. I put a box of crackers into the cabinet and sat back down, proud that I had done what she asked.

"Honey, look at the counter by the sink. What do you see?"

"The plant."

"What else do you see that you could do?"

Sorting through all of the visual stimuli to realize that washing the dishes would be a good place to start was difficult but I did it. "The plate is now dirty."

"Good. You can wash the dishes." The speech therapist had suggested that instead of correcting my sentence structure, people should repeat what I was trying to say with a prompt.

I didn't move from my chair. It takes initiative to get up and begin. "What do you need to do now?" came my mother's gentle voice.

I looked at her and then walked over to the pile of dirty dishes. I put the dishes into the sink. I turned on the water and added soap. I began to wipe the glasses, and then place them down gently to keep the clatter low to protect my ears from the clanging noise. I moved over to put the clean dishes into the drying rack. A bird landed on the deck railing outside the window. I watched the bird until it flew away and continued looking at the deck railing.

"Julie, look back at the sink and keep working." Focus. This is what my occupational therapist had called this step of the process. Turning my attention back to the plates, the water was gone, only a bit of soap remained.

I began to cry in frustration. "No good water to one mountain is gone."

My mom walked over to me to try to understand my jumbled speech. "The water drained out of the sink. Let's see what happened. Let's put the drain stopper in, and then try again. You can do it."

She noticed the soapy glasses in the drying rack and put them back into the sink to be rinsed.

"Let's list the steps in order."

"Stopper. Soap. Wash. Water done to it. Counter rack."

"And fill the sink with warm water before the soap goes in," she coached.

So many things to remember and put in order. Sequencing was the hardest part of everything. I ran the water until suds covered the plates and washed them each carefully.

I walked away and sat down at the table to open a bill. "Julie, come back over here. Completing a task is just as important as starting it."

The dishes were finally washed, rinsed, and drying in the rack. I looked at my mom. "Done it right now one time."

"Good evaluation," she said with a smile.

My occupational therapist had coached me on the six brain processes required to accomplish a task. Recognition that a job needs to be done. Initiation to begin. Sequencing the actions. Focusing on the activity. Doing the task to completion. Finally, evaluating the end result.

My mom praised me for washing the dishes while she wiped down the counters and swept the floor. I was exhausted from my efforts.

"It's time for you to rest. Let's listen to your mindfulness CD." I lay down in my loft and closed my eyes as a calming voice walked me through a visualization of a beach with the soothing sounds of the ocean. As I walked the beach, as the voice suggested, my mind returned to the frustration of the sink emptying.

"Stupid. I'm stupid. I can't even do the dishes right." In my thoughts my speech was always so clear even if my perceptions of an event were a bit distorted.

Forgetting about the CD, I remembered a day shortly before the crash. I had been at work, patrolling one of my tougher neighborhoods when I was dispatched to a robbery around the corner. I raced to the location where the victim told me a man had just taken his wallet and phone. With a quick description and direction of travel, I searched the streets as I directed backup units to set up a perimeter. While canvassing the neighborhood, a lady holding a baby came running out of a house. She said she was in the kitchen when she heard a noise in her back storage room. She had peeked into the room and saw a man hiding. My partner and I approached the back room and ordered the man to the ground at gunpoint.

"I used to catch robbers and now I can't even wash dishes right," I thought, mentally beating myself up. My mom came upstairs when she heard me crying.

"No cop even one time," I sobbed. She reminded me that I was hurt and that I would get better, a reminder I needed several times a day.

My mom said goodbye and told me that my dad would be over in a few hours. She then corrected herself and said that he would be there at 6:15 p.m. Time disorientation and an awareness of time passing had also become problems. "I'll put it on the board for you," referring to the white board where all of my reminders and daily activities were now listed.

By 9 o'clock my dad and I were almost back to the car, our evening activity coming to an end. "I'm so proud of you and how hard you worked today with Mom." I glowed at his praise as I got into the passenger seat. Riding in the car was difficult at times. My compromised depth perception made it seem that all cars were just inches from hitting us. My dad took the back roads to accommodate this after my long day.

"Do you remember where I turn?"

I pointed to the left and directed him to turn at "the red cow house."

He smiled and brought me home.

Three years later, the "red cow house" has continued to be what our family still jokingly calls barns. My speech and abilities returned and ten months after my injury I returned to my job as a police officer.

"You will get better," my mom had promised.

I have.

~Julie Sanderson

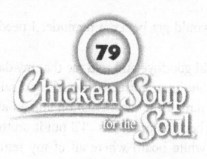

Love in the Right Place

When we are no longer able to change a situation—
we are challenged to change ourselves.
~Viktor E. Frankl

How I met her simply couldn't have been a coincidence. My car was being worked on and, as is typical for those of us with traumatic brain injury, I lost track of time until somehow, from somewhere, the memory surfaced that I had a doctor's appointment and now the car wasn't ready to drive. I decided to hitchhike.

She was driving by with her black Lab Brittney and saw this man walking, thumb out and in need. She liked my face and had a good feeling about me so she offered me a ride. It was a very lucky day.

She wasn't the only one who got a feeling that fateful day. Since my brain injury I have noticed that I "feel" people and their energy in a more spiritual and creative way. She exuded great energy and we talked so easily. I did make it to my doctor's appointment, and when I got back home I wrote in my journal, "I met this girl today who taught me how to feel. She felt good."

I had given her my card and she'd shared her phone number with me. But even though the impact she had on me was significant, I kept forgetting to call. She knew I had a brain injury and to my surprise I hadn't blown it with her after all. A couple of weeks after we'd met she called me and invited me over for lunch. It was love then. It has been ever since.

As anyone who has loved a person with a TBI knows, it isn't always easy. Most people want and need to look at the big picture of life. They easily see how things connect and are able to work through emotional issues and life events as a connected whole. That doesn't work for me or for many of us with TBI—so I had to put our love, and the parts of it that arose, in a box.

This lovely woman in my life had four younger children and also an ex-husband who was seemingly unkind. The idea of someone being cruel to this wonderful woman in my life became a near obsession for me; I wanted to fix it or rectify it somehow but I couldn't. I had to learn to deal with what had happened in the past for her or it was going to damage our relationship. I had to work hard at not getting overwhelmed. If something came up about the children's father, I mentally put that information and event in its own box. I keep a lot of things in boxes. It's a mindfulness thing where I need to look at something as a separate entity even though it's part of something larger. It takes training. I learned to do it through meditation, which has been my saving grace.

Naturally, my new friend and I tried to have a typical relationship where our lives, time and living spaces were intertwined, but it went badly. I need my things in a certain place so it keeps me organized and less apt to forget. She needed more spontaneity in her quarters. It was hard, but the love was real. We finally came to terms with my need for my own space, separate from hers. Our spaces also each had to be in their own boxes for me to manage. Luckily she is okay with remaining connected but keeping separate places.

People with TBI may need to think inside the boxes to maintain emotional health and even love at times. And those who love us may need to learn to think outside of them.

~Pete Daigle

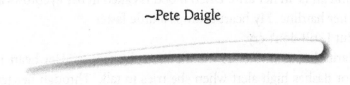

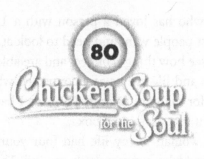

Rest Is Best

Wisely, and slowly. They stumble that run fast.
~William Shakespeare

It's a cool, rainless November evening when my cell phone rings. "Your daughter's been in a rollover car accident," the paramedic says. "We're taking her to the hospital."

For a moment, I lose my ability to think. I want to hang up the phone, get my shoes on, and get in the car. Fast. I don't cry.

As my husband drives us to the hospital, Sarita's twin brother sits in the back seat in silence. I call our other daughter at college to let her know about the accident. I am unusually calm.

At the hospital, we sit in the emergency waiting room until a social worker comes out to talk to us. "Sarita is a little disoriented and kind of confused," she says. "But that's to be expected."

She tells us we'll be able to see her as soon as they complete a CT scan and X-rays on her right arm, back, and neck. The social worker reassures us that our daughter is awake and talking. I remain calm.

Fifteen minutes later, a nurse leads us through the emergency room doors. Sarita is lying in a hospital bed with a brace around her neck and an IV in her arm. Dried blood is caked in her eyebrows and along her hairline. My heart thumps a little faster.

But I still don't cry.

Sarita bursts into tears the moment she sees us. Her heart rate monitor flashes high alert when she tries to talk. Through her tears, she asks about her friend who was driving.

"She's fine," I tell her. "You're both going to be fine." I say it with confidence, and as I do, a strange energy rushes through me.

A short time later, Sarita's scans all come back normal. But it's not the end.

"She has a concussion," the doctor says. "Her head is going to hurt for a while." He gives us instructions on her care and I try to absorb everything he says.

I help Sarita change into hospital scrubs for the ride home. We bring along an ice bag for her head and a vomit bag for her nausea. As I sit next to her in the back seat, holding tightly to her hand, she drifts in and out of sleep.

At home, I help her into bed. Then I sit down and try to read over the hospital papers the doctors gave us. Concussion: an injury that occurs when you receive a sudden blow or jolt to the head—a type of traumatic brain injury. Watch for seizures, loss of consciousness, confusion, vomiting, numbness. Rest is the best way to recovery. Limit activities. No television, no texting, no computers.

My own mind is a fog. When my husband convinces me to get some rest, I leave our bedroom door open and lie awake for a long time. How can I hear her breathe from here? Did she move? Roll over? Call for me?

I spend the following days in caretaker mode: bathing her, holding the ice pack on her head, cleaning the cuts on her forehead, and giving her pain medication. I watch the bruises on her arm deepen and spread. I ask her gently about the accident. The last thing she remembers is getting into the car.

I still don't cry.

Twelve days later, Sarita tries to go back to school. She texts me after two hours, with a headache so intense she has to close her eyes. She can't listen to her teachers. She can't look at her classmates. She comes home and sleeps. She doesn't make it through a full day that week or the next.

She tries more ibuprofen and Extra Strength Tylenol. Even though the teachers allow her extra time to complete her assignments, she starts to see her grades drop. She can't read through a whole chapter of AP biology. She complains about blurry vision. The headaches continue.

"Everybody thinks I'm fine," Sarita says.

And on the outside, it seems that way. Her cuts have almost healed. Her bruises are beginning to turn pale yellow. But her brain is another story.

More days go by. I Google everything I can about concussions. I ask friends for advice. I look for naturopathic solutions to Sarita's headache pain. Nothing changes. We both grow more frustrated.

Sarita wants her normal life back. She wants to go to school for an entire day. She wants to go out with friends and try out for the next theatrical production. And when she does, she doesn't make the cut.

"The teacher said she could see it in my eyes," Sarita says, when she gets home. "She could see that I'm not better."

I tell her there will be other plays and maybe it's for the best. Maybe she needs more time and more rest. It's not what she wants to hear.

"I didn't ask for this," she cries.

And she's right. Nobody asks to have her life put on hold. But Sarita's brain has other ideas.

That night, after I tuck her in, I finally cry. I cry for the trauma she's been through. I cry for her pain and her struggle. I cry for almost losing her.

Sarita faces each day with more strength and determination. She stays at school until the final bell rings. She plods through another chapter in her biology book. She says the headaches are not as bad as they used to be. But when she climbs into bed at 3:30 on a Wednesday afternoon, I'm not convinced.

Finally, our family doctor suggests that Sarita see a concussion specialist. The specialist asks her to rate her headaches and neck pain. He tests her ability to perform simple body movements. He asks about her mood.

Then we get his recommendation: scale it back. He suggests she only go to school half days, leaving school early on some days, starting late on others. He recommends less schoolwork, less problem solving, less thinking. Lots of nighttime sleep and daytime rest. He suggests physical therapy and maybe a walk for exercise. Some outings with friends to keep up her spirits.

"I can't scale it back," Sarita protests.

But we both know it may be the only way.

And so she rests more, thinks less. Her new glasses improve her blurry vision. The physical therapist's exercises help her neck pain. An evening with a good friend is just what she needs to put the smile back on her face. Day by day, the headaches grow less intense and less frequent.

When an entire week goes by—and then another—and Sarita stays pain free, we both laugh and cry and laugh some more. We realize that the moment Sarita listened to her brain and slowed down was the moment she began finding her way back to normal. And normal is a very sweet place to be.

—Annette Gulati

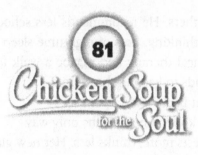

81

Every Day Is a Gift

Love always protects, always trusts, always hopes, always perseveres.
Love never fails.

~1 Corinthians 13:7-8a

I
magine how you would feel if on the inside you were the same person you have always been, but your life was totally different. You no longer have the ability to walk, talk, or eat. You no longer have any control of your own life. Insurance companies, doctors, therapists, hospitals and nursing homes no longer see you as a person, but as a statistic. You are given no prognosis.

Your diagnosis? Severe traumatic brain injury.

We'll probably never know how long my husband Henry lay crumpled in the ditch that sunny August afternoon with his motorcycle on top of him. What we do know is that a school bus driver spotted him and called 911. When the EMTs arrived, they assessed his condition and summoned a medical helicopter. Henry was Life Flighted to a university hospital in the city where we lived.

He sustained multiple facial fractures, a broken shoulder, and bruised lungs. But, in the great scheme of things, none of those injuries mattered much. Because in spite of the top-of-the-line protective helmet Henry was wearing when he crashed, he had suffered "hard brain whiplash."

He was in a deep coma. For fifteen days, I sat by Henry's bedside in the trauma unit, holding his hand and wondering whether the next breath he took would be his last. He underwent countless tests and procedures, including a craniotomy in which neurosurgeons removed part of his skull so that his brain would have room to swell.

Before he was to receive a much-needed shunt to control the fluid on his brain, Henry was transferred to another hospital while still comatose. From that hospital, Henry was sent to a nursing home where they had never had a patient with injuries as severe as his. It quickly became obvious he'd been sent there because it was assumed that sooner or later he would die from complications associated with his injuries.

Through it all, I sat by Henry's side during the day and slept next to his bed at night. I talked to him. I read to him. I sang to him. I begged him not to give up. I reminded him that he was only thirty years old and had a promising career as a graphic designer ahead of him. I fought in every way I knew how to fight to get him the care he needed.

Finally, Henry was accepted at the Patricia Neal Rehabilitation Center in Knoxville, Tennessee. I'll always believe that was the turning point in his recovery. At last, Henry had doctors and nurses who were truly knowledgeable about brain injuries. He regained the light in his eyes. He weaned himself off oxygen and was able to get his tracheostomy removed. And he received the physical, occupational, and speech therapy he desperately needed.

After three months at Patricia Neal, Henry and I finally went home. I would now be his doctor, nurse, caretaker, and therapist.

I won't pretend it's been a bed of roses since then. More than five years have passed since the motorcycle accident, and Henry and I still have a long road to recovery ahead of us. He has a feeding tube and is confined to a wheelchair. This presents problems because we live in a house that is not completely handicapped-accessible, but with the help of our friends we are working to raise funds to build one that is.

Henry understands everything and can communicate through gestures and facial expressions. He can speak a few words but is still considered nonverbal. We continue to search for a speech therapist who can help him. And because Henry's injury was to the left side of his brain, the right side of his body is very weak. He's also legally blind in his right eye.

But he's making progress every day. Slow progress, but it's steady. And that's good enough for both of us.

I teach elementary school by day and take care of Henry the rest of the time. "How do you do it?" I've been asked countless times. "Where do you find the strength?"

My answer is always the same. Love and the Lord. We make it through each day because I love Henry and he loves me, and because God is so very gracious and merciful. It's as simple as that. When we married eleven years ago, we promised to care for each other in sickness and in health, and we meant it. Every day we have together is a gift.

I've never once thought "I can't do this anymore." Not ever. But I have thought about what advice I would give other caregivers facing the many challenges of traumatic brain injury. Here are five things I would tell them:

1. Talk, laugh with, and touch your loved one just as you always have and encourage others to do the same.
2. The squeaky wheel really does get the grease. Whether you're dealing with doctors, hospitals, insurance companies, therapists, or case managers, never quit insisting upon what you know your loved one really needs.
3. Celebrate small steps. Recovery from traumatic brain injury is a marathon, not a sprint.
4. Pray without ceasing.
5. Never, never, never give up.

~Heather Roach

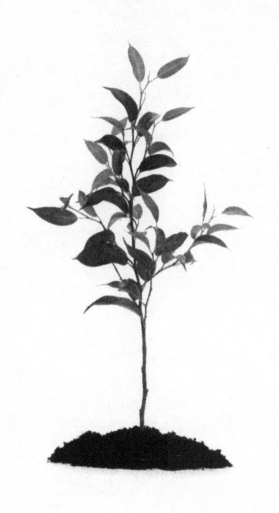

Recovering *from* Traumatic Brain Injuries

Opportunity Knocks

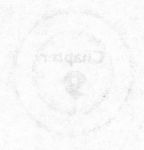

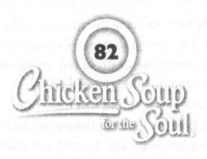

82

The Transformative Power of Words

Writing is an act of faith, not a trick of grammar.
~E.B. White

Part of the reason I wanted to edit this Chicken Soup for the Soul book on traumatic brain injury is that I believe in the healing power of words. Five years after my son Neil's traumatic brain injury, suffered at the hands of a drunk driver in a crash that killed his girlfriend, I began finally to reflect upon this horrific experience that had befallen our family. Before that, I was too busy to think too deeply about it, just putting one foot in front of the other, helping Neil heal and recover. Yes, I had journaled all the way through our ordeal and it was surely a relief to vent on the page. But to truly process an experience takes distance, both time and space. Graham Greene called it "the sliver of ice in the heart of the writer," the span needed to objectively sort out the fallout from our lives.

I first began to write short personal essays and finally published a full-length memoir. *Crash: A Mother, a Son, and the Journey from Grief to Gratitude* tells the story of Neil's TBI from my vantage point as his mother, of course, but also from my "other-side-of-the-stretcher" perspective as a doctor. People ask me if writing the book was therapeutic. In some ways the actual daily writing of the work was quite the opposite. It was like picking at scabs one after the other, refusing to let old wounds heal. Reliving the trauma on the page was painful every single time I set pencil to paper. Examining my feelings about the drunk driver, about the death of one so young, about my son's broken dreams, tested my literary mettle daily.

But now, looking back, I find that the writing was actually therapeutic after all. It gave me the opportunity to exert some control over a completely senseless situation. I could not change any aspect of the accident. I could not erase Neil's brain injury nor could I bring his girlfriend back to life. But I could control the narrative. I could not change the outcome, but I could try to make something positive come of it, by sharing our experience with others, by giving readers a more nuanced understanding of brain injury, one that considers the subtlety and diversity of its long-term effects.

A few years ago, I had the great privilege to present a writing workshop at the University of Iowa's Examined Life conference. One of my fellow presenters, Nellie Hermann, is the Creative Director of the Program in Narrative Medicine at Columbia University Medical School, which seeks to enhance medical students' patient experiences by encouraging them to write about them. Nellie had written a novel based on an event in her life that was similarly tragic to my own. She made the following observation: "We write to exert power over something we can never control. The past."

Trauma therapists have long understood this concept of using words as therapy. Often, patients with post-traumatic stress disorder are asked to record a "trauma narrative," writing down events in their lives that continue to haunt them. Then, by reading the text over and over again, something amazing and positive happens. Through words, these events eventually lose their impact. Through narrative, trauma victims regain control.

This is my hope not only for each and every one of the writers whose work is represented in this collection, but also for the many writers whose stories I have read and thought about and cried over and smiled at. I hope that the mere telling of their stories, the sharing of their narratives, helped them to gain strength and hope. Because every one of these stories, published or not, reveals courage and bravery and serves to encourage others along the way to healing.

~Carolyn Roy-Bornstein

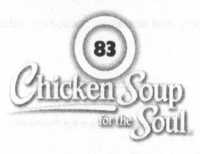

83

Adjusting Your Goals after TBI

*Patience and perseverance have a magical effect before which
difficulties disappear and obstacles vanish.*
~John Quincy Adams

My life changed completely as a result of my traumatic brain injury (TBI). I was in my third year of law school at Suffolk University in Boston. I had dreamed of becoming an attorney since I was in high school. I was a few months away from graduating and beginning my career as a trial attorney. At the time, I also worked part-time in an insurance defense law firm. I was in the top two percent of my class and made it to the quarterfinals in many trial competitions at school. My husband and I had married the summer before and were just starting our lives together.

My TBI happened as a result of a car collision. I had just left my job and was driving to Suffolk for my afternoon class. I was on a winding road heading towards the highway. I came around one bend and another driver came in the opposite direction, passed out at the wheel, crossed the median into my lane and hit me head on. I don't remember the accident, or even anything that first week, but I had the best witness in the car behind me: an FBI agent!

After the accident, I was in a coma for five days at Massachusetts General Hospital. A cranial bolt was placed in my skull to monitor the pressure in my brain. My family and friends stayed by my side waiting for me to wake up but the only person I remember visiting me at MGH was the dean of Suffolk University. I had just taken his trial practice class.

I spent the next five weeks at Spaulding Rehabilitation Hospital where I received speech, occupational and physical therapies. My biggest problems were short-term memory, word retrieval, remembering names, and loss of abstract thinking. In the beginning, I could not count from twenty to one backwards and could barely read. One of the most vivid memories I have at Spaulding was when the speech therapist showed me flash cards with pictures on them. I simply had to name what was on the card. The pictures always started with basic objects like a ball and then would become more complex. I remember always getting stuck on one card, a picture of a frog; I could not name a frog.

I improved rapidly with all the therapy at Spaulding. Before I was discharged, the lead neurologist held a team meeting so we could learn their outpatient recommendations. While I sat there, I waited for one to comment about me going back to school. I did not understand the seriousness of my injury. When friends came to visit, I told them that I was not going to graduate with my class but I would go back to school in the fall, finish up and take the bar exam in February. I waited and waited for someone to discuss my academics but no one did. Finally, I asked them about it. After a very long pause, the lead doctor stated that she did not think I would be ready for school in the fall and that maybe I would never be ready. I finally understood the reality and seriousness of my injury.

After I left this meeting, I told my family that I just could not believe this prognosis. The doctor came back to talk to me that day and recommended that if I was that resolute that perhaps after undergoing more speech therapy I might be ready in the fall to go back to school but should only take one class at a time. Despite all the sadness and shock in trying to understand my fate, I now had a long-term goal.

For the next year and a half, I participated in outpatient speech therapy at a local hospital. I did go back to school, and with the help of my speech therapist, took my classes one at a time. I would often bring my law school books to therapy and read her the cases that I needed to comprehend. I would then explain to her what I had just read. She would also review writing assignments to make sure that my ideas flowed. I didn't do as well with my classes as before my TBI but I did complete them. Two years later, I finally graduated cum laude and took the bar exam. With extra time accommodations, I was able to pass the bar on my first try.

I also have epilepsy because of my TBI. I began having partial complex seizures right after the accident. Periodically, I would have a grand mal seizure and I had one status epileptic seizure, a continuous, unremitting seizure lasting longer than five minutes. I have been on many anti-seizure drugs and have had to live with many side effects but still do not have complete seizure control. Almost eight years after my accident, I chose to have an operation to help, a left temporal lobe resection. My operation is considered a success because I now have just one or two partial complex seizures per month instead of a dozen, although I still have to take multiple anti-seizure medications and probably will for the rest of my life.

I had to go through a lot to come to terms with the reality that I am not able to practice law but can use some of the skills to move on to another career. I found a way to use my talents working at the Brain Injury Association of Massachusetts (BIA-MA). At the BIA-MA, I helped to implement the Ambassador Program. I recruit Ambassadors, either survivors or family members, to share their knowledge and personal insight into brain injury and to make a seamless link between prevention and real life examples. I assist Ambassadors to write their awe-inspiring stories. The Ambassadors then present their stories to a variety of audiences, including at local civic groups, businesses, and medical facilities. Finally, I am using my legal skills to implement a better Advocacy Program for our organization for TBI survivors. I am trying to make things better in a small way for the brain injury community.

~Kelly Buttiglieri

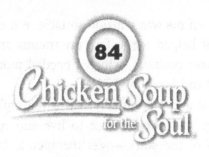

84

Writing

Write injuries in dust, benefits in marble.
~Benjamin Franklin

My husband and I had been married for three months. It was 1990 and life was good. I was working at a shopping mall in Southern California. One evening after work, as I pulled out of the mall parking lot, my car stalled in the middle of the road. A city bus hit me, leaving me near death.

I was in a coma and had brain surgery. My brain was injured so badly that the doctors thought I would be paralyzed; they also said I would never be the same, never think clearly again. But I surprised them when I moved my hands and then eventually stood up and with help, began to walk. In a few months I was able to walk on my own. However, the struggle to regain my mental health as well as my balance and coordination took another ten years. Speech was also a major difficulty for me at first. My words slurred. I had trouble finding words at all.

As I recovered, I began to write. The act itself helped me to sort out the scattered words in my mind. Putting my thoughts on paper also helped me deal with the severe symptoms of post-traumatic stress disorder that seemed to get worse with the years.

Recovery from traumatic brain injury has been unbelievably intense, but also incredibly deepening and spiritual. At the beginning, recovery focused on my physical limitations. I still have extensive trouble with memory, speech and PTSD. The emotional toll my limitations took on me was a major obstacle. But even at my worst, I kept writing. It helped me to face my trauma and work through it. Nurturing these positives, which I needed more than life itself, healed my mind and eased my PTSD.

My husband and I eventually had seven children. Their love gave me courage and perseverance to live and recover. And writing—regardless of the story—was therapeutic for my heart and mind. Journaling finally grew into novels, leading to my return to college thirteen years after my accident. The more I studied, the clearer and more organized my thoughts became. The research I did for my novels helped me in my coursework, but my recovery while in college has become more defined. My thinking has grown sharper than it would have ever been before I had the brain injury and recovery. I am grateful to have gained the strength and courage to recover from such an insurmountable injury. Now I have the courage to share what I've written with others, and though my memory still suffers, it's a small price to pay for the bounty I have received.

~Justine Johnston Hemmestad

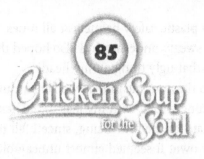

85

What I Learned from a Severe TBI

*I've often said there's nothing better for the inside of a man
than the outside of a horse.*

~Ronald Reagan

Tied down to a hospital bed, I moaned and cried, trying to wiggle free. "Haaaalooooo! Haaaaaaloooooooo! Anybody?" when suddenly my mother leaned over me. What was she doing here? Shouldn't she be in Germany? And where was I anyway? This didn't make sense at all!

"The doctors want to transfer you to a different hospital, one that specializes in your kind of injury. Is that okay with you?" my mother asked me in our native language. I nodded, not even knowing what "my kind of injury" was, and drifted back into unconsciousness, a place I much preferred to be.

Weeks later, I learned that Anatole, the horse I had galloped and jumped over hurdles one morning at the track, took a misstep, stumbled, and fell, which left me unconscious with a severe traumatic brain injury. To my relief, Anatole was unharmed and continued his racing career successfully. I was happy for him, but I also wondered: What about *my* racing career?

My shaved head and long scars were evidence of the craniotomy the neurosurgeon had performed to give my brain room to swell and hopefully avoid more damage. For that reason, I was required to wear one of those ugly plastic safety helmets at all times. Not only did my head get hot and sweaty underneath, I also hoped that no one would ever see me with that ugly thing on my head.

And why did they put me into a wheelchair during the daytime? Was there something wrong with my legs too? Then again, I appreciated the wheelchair for the time being, since I felt too weak to stand or to walk on my own. It seemed almost unbearable to sit up all day. All I wanted was to lie down and rest, logging out for a while, hoping that the next time I woke up, my old life would be back: filled with laughter, friends, horses, and the racetrack, with all its excitement.

Because of terrible coughing attacks accompanied with gasping for air, breathing wasn't easy either. I had a breathing tube in my throat, which looked and felt creepy. More than just once a day, the filter would fall off and needed to be screwed back on. It irritated me every time that there was this thing that could be screwed back onto the front of my throat.

The tracheostomy, where the doctor had made a cut underneath my vocal cords into the windpipe to allow air to enter my lungs, needed to be revised because of growing scar tissue. This time the doctor disconnected my vocal cords to prevent that from happening again. That procedure shut me up for six weeks. Not even a whisper came out of my mouth. Left with my own dreadful thoughts, pen and paper became a necessity to make communication possible. I waited for the day the doctor would give me my voice back and I would be able to ask for some clarity about my situation.

After the craniotomy, a bump had formed on the left side of my head. It kept swelling and jiggled uncontrollably with every movement. In another surgery the neurosurgeon put burr holes into the bump to drain the collected fluid out. My head shrank back to its original size. Great! Now my ugly safety helmet fit again!

After all of the medical intervention, as well as five months of speech, occupational, and physical therapy, I regained strength and balance. The missing piece of my skull was replaced. I traded the safety helmet for a wool cap. I now looked more like a cancer patient waiting for my hair to grow back. Day after day, week after week, and month after month, I searched for someone to blame, before I finally gave in and believed that God came through and protected me for a reason. Now the more important question became: Where did I go from there?

Despite my physical and mental recovery, I had turned into a complete wreck emotionally. Returning to where I had been didn't seem possible, or so I was told. Due to steroids and inactivity, I had gained over forty pounds, which prevented my reentry into the world of horse racing. The excess weight stopped me from doing what I loved most and left me feeling unworthy and unattractive. Suicide as a complete checkout and the final solution for my misery sounded more and more appealing.

But something inside me wasn't yet ready to call it quits. I surely wanted to ride horses again, feel the sunshine warming my skin, breathe in the fresh morning air, and show the world I still had something to contribute. I channeled all of my energy to find a new path. A friend recommended a career as a therapeutic riding instructor. But was it possible to start a new career in that field? And how would I get there?

This time my four-legged therapists helped me find the answer. In equine-assisted therapy, an activity that included my old and my new worlds, the horses gave me the idea that there was plenty of room in between, and that it was okay for me to not already be exactly where I wanted to be. They showed me how important it was to stay calm, focused and enjoy the journey. And most of all they reminded me once again to live in the present moment, since yesterday was nothing more than a memory, while tomorrow was nothing but a dream.

With determination and focus, I was able to stay productive. With time, newly learned patience, the ability to take life day by day, and the assurance of being perfectly guided, I would conquer the mountain that, at first, seemed too high to climb. There was so much more to learn from horses than just enjoying the thrill of going fast.

~Vanessa Friedrich

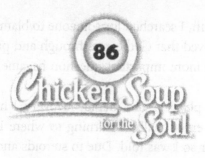

Silver Lining

Accept the things to which fate binds you, and love the people with whom fate brings you together, but do so with all your heart.

~Marcus Aurelius

If only I knew ten years ago what I know now. Like all high school seniors applying to college, I wrote quite a few essays. While most of the questions were quite forgettable, one still sticks in my mind ten years later. The question, "Explain the saying every cloud has a silver lining," wasn't easy for me to answer at the time, and I'm sure I gave a hypothetical answer since, as a fortunate eighteen-year-old kid I hadn't experienced many "clouds" in my life.

I got into college and received my diploma in May 2006 at the age of twenty-three. Two months later, on July 4, I made the awful decision to drive after drinking. As a result, I crashed my car, sustained a traumatic brain injury, and spent three months in the hospital.

After my discharge from Spaulding Rehab Hospital in Boston, I moved in with my parents in Cape Neddick. Four days a week I received tremendous rehabilitation services at Portsmouth Regional Hospital. As my rehab became less time-consuming I slipped into a deep depression. Even though I had an unbelievable support network of family and friends, I felt as if I were an outcast and a burden. I decided I wanted to start volunteering.

I contacted the Seacoast's United Way branch, but couldn't seem to find the right opportunity. Then I remembered being told about the Krempels Center in Portsmouth. The center runs a community-based day program for adults living with acquired brain injury from trauma, tumor or stroke. It struck me as the perfect opportunity: to work with a group that I was also a member of. I called and spoke with a staff member who told me to come in on Monday, Wednesday or Friday to check out the program. My dad dropped me off, nervous about leaving me, struggling to walk with one side of my body greatly impaired. I was nervous, too, but happy to have something new to do.

My plan of volunteering took a dramatic turn as I sat in on the program's morning community meeting in which announcements were made and the day's schedule was explained. I was amazed to see the diverse group of brain-injured individuals. Everyone was smiling, conversing and seemed genuinely glad to be together. This was what I had been missing out on; I had survived, but I wasn't living.

Instead of volunteering, I became a member and still continue to be after three years. I am inspired every time I leave the center. I remember leaving that day, feeling part of the world again; in retrospect, I had found my silver lining.

~Jim Scott

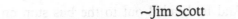

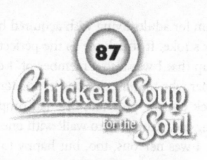

Unstoppable

Patience and tenacity are worth more than their weight of cleverness.
~Thomas Huxley

C hris and I married in our twenties. On our wedding day, we imagined our lives would be wonderful, full of fun, kids, and memories galore. But instead, we've traveled a journey we never could have imagined.

On a crystal clear blue-sky day in June, Chris softly kissed me as I slowly awakened from my slumber. "The kids are watching *Sesame Street*," he whispered. And he headed out to the bus stop on our corner.

The screech of brakes shook me from my sleepy fog. Immediately, I heard screaming. "Someone call an ambulance!"

I scrambled downstairs, thoughts racing. Chris would be the first one to call for help. I didn't hear the bus go by. Panic edged into my mind. I glanced at my little girls watching TV; they were fine. I pushed open the front door and peered through the screen. A small crowd stood over a body in the street.

"Is it a man?"

A stranger looked up and nodded.

"Does he have a moustache?"

Another nod.

I flew out the door.

My husband had been hit by a truck. He was lying in the street, semi-conscious, blood pooled around his head. The blare of sirens grew louder.

"Chris... Chris. It's me. It's Elise, your wife. Hold on, honey. You're going to be okay."

The EMTs rushed to Chris's side, checked his vital signs, then quickly but gingerly lifted him into the ambulance.

"You'll have to follow behind," they told me.

I ran to the neighbors', blurting an explanation, begging them to watch my children. A young woman beckoned me to the transport vehicle. We trailed the ambulance to the trauma hospital, sirens screaming, lights flashing.

In shock, I cried, begged, "Please God, please let Chris live."

We careened into the emergency room entrance as Chris lost consciousness. Medical personnel ushered me into a small spare private waiting room where I was asked to sign scary documents detailing procedures I didn't understand.

How could this be? How could I be in a hospital with my husband on the brink of death?

Suddenly, our dear friend, a developmental pediatrician, burst into the waiting room. Instead of his usual commute, he was heading to a meeting and just happened to be in the area when his wife paged him. And now, here he was, explaining every update, every intricacy of what was happening. He injected some clarity and peace into this nightmare.

Chris survived the surgery, the first huge hurdle.

A sweet quiet nurse in scrubs entered the waiting room where now many family members gathered. "You can see your husband now."

Fear shook me to my core. "Your husband is stable, but he is unconscious and bruised." The nurse tried to prepare me in a whisper. Gauze covered his head like a mummy. Intravenous lines led to beeping, whirring machines. His face was black and blue, both eyes purple, swollen shut.

Chris remained in an induced coma for three days. All we could do was wait and see. Dazed, I drifted through days and nights, staying by my husband's side. As he came to, he didn't know who I was. He didn't remember his three children. He communicated mostly through unintelligible mumbles and gestures. What lay ahead?

Eventually Chris was moved out of the ICU to a general med-surg floor. There he got basic therapy, scrawling his name, speaking in scrambled sentence fragments, wide-eyed with confusion.

After a week, Chris was moved to a rehabilitation facility. My once healthy independent husband was now totally dependent on others to care for him. Yet he was determined and courageous in the face of huge obstacles.

He worked tirelessly at relearning everything—how to talk, walk, write, bathe, feed himself. When I went to visit in the evenings, Chris grimaced. "This is really hard." He was absolutely exhausted after every long day of grueling workouts, constantly pushing himself to reach every single bar his speech, physical, and occupational therapists set for him.

After several weeks, Chris moved back home. I was terrified. What if he slipped in the shower? What if he wandered out when I wasn't watching? What if he fell down the stairs? What if he hit his head?

He continued daily trips to rehab. Our neighbors, friends, families, even strangers pitched in to help us. Dinners were delivered to our doorstep. A neighbor transported Chris to and from rehab every single day. Offers for help with the kids were constant. Cards and prayers poured in from literally all over the world.

Soon it was time for Chris to return to his job in marketing. It was too early, according to his rehab therapists, but his office insisted he at least try a part-time reentry. It was almost more than I could bear to see Chris standing back out on that street corner where he was hit, waiting for the bus again. But he was unstoppable. At times Chris got depressed, felt useless and discouraged. But he'd just push through.

One evening, Chris returned home from work. His eyes were hollow, shoulders stooped in defeat. He could no longer do his job. We sat in our backyard and cried. What would happen next?

Within a few days, Chris reached out to some old contacts and began teaching poetry workshops around the state. They seemed to go okay. Each day, I held my breath in fear. What if Chris got confused or lost? What if someone was impatient or mean to him?

I was astounded at the bravery Chris mustered for every assignment. Oh, there were panicked calls from time to time. Chris got lost... or worried he didn't do a good job. But every time, he would get up again the next morning, walk out that door, and face the new day fearlessly, with all its complications and possibilities.

Chris had earned his MFA in Poetry from Columbia University years before. Ready for the next challenge, he marched up to the local university and applied for an adjunct professor position. Again, I paced and wrung my hands in anxiety, waiting to hear. Chris was excited and confident. He got the job! This was unbelievable... a miracle!

Within a couple of years at the university, Chris decided to go for his doctorate in education. What? This was just crazy. Not only did it seem impossible, but we couldn't afford to send Chris to school. Our oldest daughter was entering college, too. But my husband just smiled. "I'll just take the next step and apply."

He got in. Exciting, but we couldn't afford it. I figured it was a done deal. Then, one day late in August, a couple of weeks before classes started, there was a letter laid out on the dining room table.

"Congratulations! We are offering you an assistantship to cover your tuition..." It was a full scholarship.

It has been twenty years since the accident. I knew when I married Chris that he was a good man: smart, loyal, kind, strong. But I never could have imagined his tenacity, confidence mixed with humility, and unwavering resolve. He is my hero. He may be brain-injured, but he has accomplished more than I could have ever imagined possible.

~Elise Daly Parker

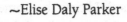

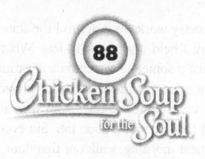

Accidental Destiny

Children are the anchors that hold a mother to life.

~Sophocles

As a restaurant manager, my days off were few and far between. But tonight I had a rare evening off and I couldn't get out the door fast enough. Just as I was leaving work I heard my assistant call out, "Phone for you, Cecile."

As tempted as I was to pretend I was not there and have them take a message, I took the call. My assistant handed me the phone and he knew right away something was wrong. "Hello, Cecile speaking," I said, forcing cheer into my voice.

The voice on the other end of the line was familiar, but my father's tone was an unfamiliar mix of panic and worry. "Hello, Cecile. Papa here. I'm so glad I caught you. I can't seem to get through on your cell phone." Suddenly, my throat tightened; something was wrong. Mom did the calling in our house, not Papa. He would come on the phone after Mom and I chatted, usually at the end of the conversation so he could say, "So good to hear your voice, Sunshine. I love you!"

"What's wrong, Papa?" I demanded, knowing he tries to sugarcoat things for his little girl.

"I have some news. Are you sitting down?" he said with a choke in his voice. At that instant, I knew that something horrible had happened. Our family unit of three was a solid triangle. We were a team, and little did I know that team was going to become very important and much stronger.

He barely choked out the words, "It's your mother. There was an accident. They don't really know what the damage is, but she hasn't woken up yet."

The room started spinning. My mind was struggling to piece it together. My knees felt weak. My assistant immediately recognized that this was not just a work phone call and something had gone terribly wrong. I felt so helpless and far away.

I began driving as the sun rose. Thirteen hours to the Kingston hospital and I think I made it in eleven. There was nowhere else I wanted to be. I didn't tell my father I was driving, because I knew that would worry him. I just kept calling him and asking for updates.

Finally I raced through the emergency room doors. "My mom is here; she was hit by a car," I gasped. There was no hesitation from the young girl at the desk as she instantly jumped to her feet. "You must be Wendy's daughter," she said and led me into a small room where my mother lay hooked to tubes and machines. My father was sitting beside the bed, his head buried in hands.

The moment I entered, my mom stirred. "Cecile?" Then her voice trailed off and went silent.

My father's head jolted up with the sound of her voice; he had been waiting for her to speak since the accident the day before. He stood up and looked at me; tears streamed down his face as he squeezed me. "God bless you. I knew you would come. I knew you would come."

I tried to share his optimism. I expected bad, but this was worse. Most of her ribs were fractured; she had a broken leg and a back injury. It was the brain injury that changed my mom; it transformed and challenged our family in ways I had never dreamed it could. Getting her out of the hospital was only the beginning. Her rehabilitation included speech therapy, dozens of tests and multiple therapist appointments.

The change in her personality and mental stability was the hardest to grasp. I felt that I had lost my best friend. Our parent/child roles were reversed. My mom had spent her life as an entrepreneur who also volunteered teaching disadvantaged children theatre arts and drama. She still had a strong fighting spirit inside her, and even on those days when her mind was clouded with pain and confusion, determination was there.

For the first two years, I traveled back and forth and I pored over the latest research on brain injury. At first, it was like a foreign language to me. Gradually, I began to not only decipher the information, but I became fascinated by this amazing organ that is the brain. I began devouring medical journals and studying case reports of traumatic brain injuries. The more I researched, the more amazed I became. One day, like a cloudburst, it came to me. This is what I wanted to devote my life to.

Suddenly, college was making a lot of sense. I applied to university, was accepted, and I am now in my third year and in the top ten percent of my class. I continue to manage my mom's ongoing care, and rarely does a day go by that she doesn't exercise her brain with some brain games that research shows improve cognitive function and memory.

Support from the community is so important. In fact, when I discovered there was no brain injury support group in my part of the country, I made some inquiries. One step led to another, and I am now helping to launch a support group in my city and becoming the area's contact for the Brain Injury Association of Canada.

It has been just over five years and I am very content with the life I have chosen. My family is closer than ever and my mom is still my best friend.

~Cecile Proctor

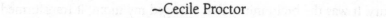

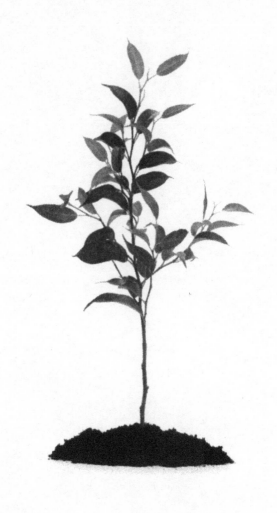

Chapter 10

Recovering *from* Traumatic Brain Injuries

Making a Difference

Chapter

10

Recovering from Traumatic Brain Injuries

Making a Difference

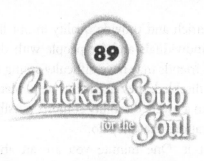

Disabilities Can Teach Us How to Live

It matters if you just don't give up.

~Stephen W. Hawking

At first it can be difficult to imagine living the rest of your life with a brain injury. As a neurologist and medical director of a rehabilitation hospital, I see many people with brain injuries, some mild and many much worse. I frequently hear my able-bodied friends say that they don't think they could live with a severe disability. But they are viewing an uncertain future through the prism of their current situation. For the last forty years, I have worked with people with brain injuries. Both they and their families have taught me a great deal about how to live and how to move forward in their new lives.

My patients are terrific examples that should allay my friends' unfounded fears. Immediately after their injuries, survivors may be unable to move their arms or legs, breathe without the help of a ventilator, or perform the most intimate routines without someone's help. But, as time passes, and with the help of rehabilitation, family, and friends, they go on to live in "their now." While it is not an easy path to travel, it is one that millions of people take every day.

At one time or another, all of us ask ourselves what represents quality in our lives. On a bad day, it may seem like there is little quality, while other days are filled with great joy. The truth is that most of the things that enrich and provide quality in our lives are the same for able-bodied individuals and for people with disabilities. But at first, able-bodied friends may have difficulty seeing it that way. If you or a loved one is disabled, they need your help. Many people assume that someone with a severe disability couldn't possibly have the same dreams and aspirations that they do.

Think about it. One minute you are an able-bodied young woman, strong and leading a normal life. Then, in a split second a car accident leaves you severely disabled. Did your dreams, aspirations and the things that brought you joy change? No, the dreams are there, but the ability to achieve them is more difficult. You may need to make some adjustments, but it is important that you maintain active goals.

When people think about living with a severe disability, they focus on the physical aspects of the disability. Healthcare professionals are quite good at helping people compensate for their physical impairments, but the real challenge is in areas we rarely think about.

Say you have a group of friends who will go out to lunch or meet you for a cup of coffee at Starbucks. Now, after your brain injury, the pool of people willing to have that cup of coffee may have narrowed. Inside your head, you may feel like the same person, but your friends may have a hard time figuring out how to interact with you. Your peer group initially visits you, but over time they may stop calling you. This is an opportunity to be the teacher, and to educate them about your disability and how to maintain a relationship. You have to become more proactive in reaching out to those friends. Make a list of your friends and call them once a week. Invite them to come over to your house or to go out for that cup of coffee. Don't wait for them to call you.

There is a great deal of attention given to maintaining social networks for the elderly, but the same is true for people with disabilities. You and your family must make the extra effort to maintain a social network that may now, hopefully, include other brain injury survivors and their families. At first you may resist interacting with other people with disabilities, but they have walked in your shoes and will have invaluable advice.

There is another opportunity to form rewarding relationships. At work, you interacted with your peer group, developed social relationships and found ways to get recognition. You may not be able to return to your previous job or any kind of work, but you will still benefit from interacting with other people. Think about starting out as a volunteer. You might even contact the hospital where you went for your rehabilitation. It is a place where both you and the staff will feel comfortable dealing with your brain injury.

Don't become insulated in your own disability. How can you prevent this? When people ask how they can help, be candid. Early on, when you are in the hospital, you and your family may not need their help. But when you get home you may need transportation or just someone to chat with. Let people know that they should volunteer again when you get home. I know families that make out a schedule and ask people if they can write in their name for a specific date and time. How about Tuesdays from 2 to 4 p.m.?

Finally, we all think about our future prospects. No matter how good our lives are at the moment, we like to think about our next vacation, going out to dinner, or something as simple as our plans with our children for the next weekend—maybe the beach.

Catastrophic injuries and illnesses may bring a sudden halt to an individual's or family's plans. Once the initial part of rehabilitation is complete, we as your rehabilitation providers need to provide you with a "prescription" that will allow you to make a successful transition into areas that give you an optimistic future. It is not always easy to align your future with your abilities. Try to make plans that give you something to look forward to, no matter how small or trivial it may seem. It may be as simple as planning to go out to dinner and a movie while putting off your goal of going to Disney World until next year.

These are not just lessons for the disabled, but for all of us. It should not take a disability or illness for us to recognize the importance of our family, social and work relationships. Living with a disability forces us to address the priorities in life that we all take for granted.

~Richard C. Senelick, MD

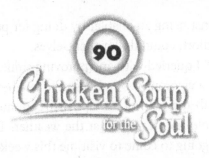

90

The Art Speaks

The aim of art is not to represent the outward appearance of things, but their inward significance.

~Aristotle

When the beautiful young woman rolled into my art room for the first time, her angry frown was the first hint that I had my work cut out for me. From reading her chart I knew that Janet's injuries were from a car accident. She could not walk, was unable to speak, and had partial use of only one hand.

So how was she going to create art?

Without hesitation Janet halted her electric wheelchair at the table where drawing paper, markers, pencils and crayons were already set out. She reached her shaky hand for a marker and began to scribble on the paper. Each stroke grew more impassioned and uncontrolled.

For the next fifteen minutes her feelings of intense anger screamed out from the saturated paper. Panting with exhaustion, she sat back in her chair and looked up at me with a huge grin.

Part of my role as an art psychotherapist in the residential TBI treatment facility was to provide art materials and methods that would help my patients creatively restore a sense of self-worth. I felt fortunate that my master's degree in art therapy education included interventions for and an understanding of physical, psychological, neurological and speech deficits. I also knew it was important for me to guard against being an enabler by doing for patients like Janet what they, with effort, could do for themselves.

"Feel better?" I queried with an approving smile.

She nodded a vigorous yes and began to laugh when she looked at her paper. With the help of an alphabet communications board, she laboriously told me, "I'm mad at the weather. The snow means my family is not going to come to visit me this weekend."

Over the following months of her stay at the rehab center, Janet learned she could safely give voice to her frustrations through her artwork and explored new ways to feel successful.

Because Janet's father died while she was in a coma, some of her anger was related to grieving his death. Family members provided photos that she used to meticulously complete a collage of her early life and special memories with her dad. She also composed a poem in his honor as the centerpiece for the collage. The artwork she created not only gave her a sense of accomplishment, it provided her a way to "speak" about his death and get some closure.

Many of my patients, like Janet, had poor motor coordination or use of only one hand. What would take me minutes to draw, took them several sessions to complete. Because of speech deficits, they drew what they wanted to say.

For my patients surviving and thriving with TBI, art is a form of self-expression without concern for aesthetic quality. With paint and paper, in color, texture, and form, their art becomes the words they cannot say, the emotions that cannot be expressed. But each of them shows me something larger: they are revealing to me a world of patience, tenacity and fortitude that I can only one day hope to attain for myself.

~Maryanne Higley Hamilton, MAT, ATR

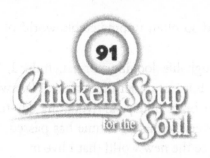

91

Living a Life of Purpose after Brain Injury

I slept and dreamt that life was service. I awoke and saw that life was service.
I acted and behold, service was joy.
~Rabindranath Tagore

As I lay sprawled out on Main Street, my body broken from being struck by a car, the last thing I envisioned was that this would be a turning point in my life.

"Call 911! Call 911!" screamed a voice as I drifted in and out of consciousness on the roadside. As I was unable to move, a passerby entered my field of vision, tears streaming down her face. I thought of my wife Sarah. Minutes earlier I had said, "Goodbye" and, "I love you," as I hopped on my bike. If I was about to die, I wanted to hear her voice one last time.

I called out her phone number, over and over. A passerby used his cell phone to call her. "Your husband has been in a bad cycling accident and the ambulance is taking him to a trauma center." Like me, only a few miles away, she wondered if I was going to die. As I lay there surrounded by first responders and other emergency personnel, pain coursing through my body, I thought that my life was truly about to end.

Though not in the way I envisioned, my life did indeed end that day. For it was on November 11, 2010 that a teenage driver broadsided me while I was out on my daily cycle ride. I was catapulted into the new and so often unpredictable world of traumatic brain injury.

I walk through life looking normal. Indeed, TBI is called "a silent epidemic." But just under the surface, I live with a hidden disability. Like other brain injury survivors, my day-to-day challenges seemed at first overwhelming. As time has passed, however, I have learned to embrace the new world that I live in.

Like so many others who share my brain-injured fate, challenges abound. My memory is a fraction of what it was in my pre-injury life. A brain injury-induced speech impediment means that I now stutter and stammer when I'm tired. My ability to discern the passage of time, as I once knew it, is gone.

So much of the "old David" did indeed die on that cold November day.

If the story ended there, nothing but tragedy would have come from my accident. But so often, from death springs new life. Fate had other plans for me. My first year as a brain injury survivor was the most difficult year of my life. Small tasks required Herculean effort. As my broken bones healed, my secret hope was that my brain injury would heal as well. I mourned the loss of my old life. Nothing made sense anymore and a new person was living in my old body.

Out of this season of suffering, new life lessons were learned. And ever so slowly, I started to regain my footing as a true survivor. From deep within the wellspring of my soul, a new strength and sense of purpose began to become clear.

Unlike so many others who had lost much of their voice, my voice became clear. Disinhibition, so common among brain injury survivors, became my friend. I had a story to tell and it was time to let the world know that life after a brain injury was possible. And I did what many over-achievers do: I set my sights high. How high? Most of my second year was spent writing a book about my experience as a survivor. Driven by some inner need to chronicle my experience, I set pen to paper and wrote.

Writing a book is a colossal undertaking in and of itself. As a brain injury survivor, to see it through to completion and successful publication let me know that almost anything is possible and that the biggest limits I have in my ongoing recovery are those limits that I put on myself.

Survivors from around the world have reached out to me and said thank you. Almost weekly, I read comments like, "you have said what I am unable to say." My experience as a brain injury survivor has made me uniquely helpful, as I understand the struggles others face, not because I read about them, but because I live them daily. I have been blessed with a circle of other survivors as I now co-facilitate a local brain injury support group. Having been a part of this group for several years, it has been such a gift to watch new members come in, to see them feel the love and acceptance of other survivors, and to move forward with a level of courage that so often inspires me.

And life goes on, as it inevitably does. Regularly, I ask myself what I can do to continue to help others. The circle grows wider still as so many family members have shared that my words have helped them to better understand what their loved ones, as brain injury survivors, are facing.

Someone much wiser than me once said that the world would be an amazing place if everyone who overcame a hardship spent time helping others who have the same hardship. Though I will never have my old life back, helping others has added a sense of real purpose to my life. During that extraordinarily painful first year, I am glad that suicide was not my fate, though I pondered it. I am grateful that God has given me the strength to persevere, as there really is a meaningful life that can be achieved after a brain injury.

One of my favorite prayers is the Prayer of Saint Francis. In this powerful prayer, Saint Francis says it is "better to forgive than to be forgiven… it is in giving that we receive." I have adapted one line of this prayer since my injury.

"It is in healing that we are healed."

And so my life has become. I do my best to help others affected by brain injury. I do all I can to help them heal. And somewhere in this miraculous process, I am healed.

For that, I am forever grateful.

~David A. Grant

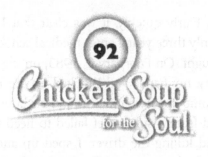

Brain Drain

*The secret of change is to focus all of your energy, not on fighting the old,
but on building the new.*

~Socrates

When I was a teenager, life was complicated. To quiet my mind and impose some structure on my life, I dove into the world of math and physics. I loved the foundational meta-galactic language and the beauty and finesse of formulas. The big picture transported me away from the conflict in my life circumstances, and eventually led me to NASA's Jet Propulsion Lab.

I loved the "little city"; I finally felt safe and secure, appreciated for what I had to offer, and never judged for what I could not provide. I reveled at my post in the spectrometry lab, some days getting lost in the tasks at hand and rarely thinking beyond my workspace. Eventually, though, the director encouraged me to move beyond the walls of the compound into a world populated by people my own age: college. I was terrified.

Months later, I had found a new comfort zone, pre-med at UCSD's Revelle College. I fully immersed myself in all that I loved, consuming calculus, physics, and biology. I added classes in dance and drama to round out my schedule, and it was there that I met the man I would later marry.

As with all things in my life, I moved through at warp speed. I juggled my courses, roommates, and relationship, trying to find a healthy balance. Fairly quickly, it was clear that I would graduate early and after only three years, enter medical school.

Or so I thought. On February 5, 1983, on the afternoon of our engagement party, my fiancé and I picked up our cake and headed to my parents' home. Just two miles from their house, a driver trying to enter the road from a side street failed to heed the stop sign. In an effort to avoid killing the driver, I sped up and moved around the front of his vehicle. I successfully avoided the T-bone, but when I braked, my Mustang spun out of control. Nearly three blocks later, we crashed into a parked car. Even though I'd been strapped in with a five-point harness, the impact caused me to burst through the seat belt and lurch forward towards the front windshield. Hitting the steering wheel, I was then launched into the back, striking the rear window. After impact, I was again thrown forward, coming to rest as my head struck the driver door.

Everything was a blur. The owner of the vehicle called my parents and they came to get us. Someone called a tow truck, and we went on to the party. One of the guests at the engagement party was a doctor and I was given muscle relaxants and a glass of wine. I remember nothing of the party or much of the time that followed. Just days later, my parents loaned us a car and we returned to college.

I remember the day I returned to class and looked up as my professor wrote integrals on the black board. It was in that moment that I knew something was terribly wrong. None of the scribbles made any sense to me—even the calculus concepts seemed like a foreign tongue rather than the language I had come to love. Frightened, I rushed off to my next class—only to find that the formulas of physics were equally strange to my injured brain. Panicked, I returned home trying to understand what was happening to me. I tried to sleep, remembering that someone had told me that rest would help me heal. But sleep was filled with nightmares of the accident replaying over and over again.

The following day, I returned to campus by way of a tree-lined road. As the sun flickered through the trees rhythmically, I started to feel nauseous. I pulled to the side of the road to vomit, growing very concerned about this new symptom. By the day's end, I found myself unable to express my thoughts accurately—struggling to produce rudimentary language. It was then that I made the decision to seek help.

The following morning, a nurse practitioner examined me and ordered a CT scan. She evaluated my symptoms and proclaimed that I'd experienced whiplash and a bad concussion. She suggested that with rest, it was likely that my symptoms would abate and that things would return to normal. After all, I was only nineteen.

But they didn't. Very soon, it became clear that medical school was no longer in my future. Math and physics were like ghosts in my wounded brain—I could still remember how much I loved them, but their elements were nowhere to be seen. They literally meant nothing to me. The dean recommended that I consider another big picture science in order to complete my education and keep moving forward. I changed my major to psychology and began to grieve.

Over time, I uploaded new language to manage the minimal aphasia that resulted from my brain injury. Six hours into my day, words would begin to fade and I would find myself mute, seeing the images of words in my mind, but unable to generate speech. Eventually, as I learned more language, the duration of fluency grew and I could make it through an entire day of class. But, when tired or stressed, I would again find myself mute.

I wish that the aphasia was all that resulted from the accident, but time revealed other, much more extensive impairments. Unfortunately for me, my physicians failed to speak with one another, so all of my symptoms were considered separately—resulting in hormone destabilization, a sleep disorder, the inability to control body temperature and cholesterol, full body spasms resembling grand mal seizures and eventually repeated pregnancy losses. By the time my symptoms were considered together, I had endured far more than the loss of a promising career.

Despite the blow I was dealt, I didn't give up. I threw myself into the development of new lingual and cognitive strategies. I designed and implemented alternate career plans. I went to graduate school and successfully earned both masters and doctoral degrees—all with a brain drained of its contents and uploaded anew. After licensure, I found myself working more and more often with other trauma survivors, eventually specializing in the field. And, after almost a decade, I found an endocrinologist who listened to all my seemingly unrelated symptoms and told me that I was going to be okay. She contacted a neurologist she'd worked with many times, and scheduled an evaluation. Unlike any of the other doctors I'd seen, he was able to evoke the symptoms, label and define the affected areas of the brain, then ordered the MRI to document the damage.

I began a regimen of medications and in three months' time, felt better than I had in sixteen years. My sleep and mood improved drastically, my hormones stabilized, my cholesterol returned to near normal levels, and for the first time in many years, I realized that recovery from brain injury could be achieved. Sometimes my patients still have to finish my sentences at the end of the day, but it's a small price to pay for what could have cost me my life.

~Sage de Beixedon Breslin, Ph.D

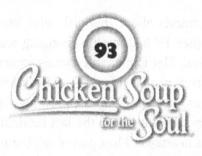

93

Seeds of Benefit

Every adversity, every failure, every heartache carries with it the seed of an equal or greater benefit.

~Napoleon Hill

I can't say I'm glad the accident happened to me—not totally. Of course I'd rather have had a life that was less of a struggle, one where I wouldn't have to fight so much with organization or be overwhelmed with terrible fatigue. However, there's a part of me that is glad it did change my life. I'm not saying I was a bad person before the car accident that destroyed so much of my brain, but I was vaguely indifferent to people who suffered. I'd think, "That's sad, but what can I do?" Then I'd go on with my life, disconnected from those suffering people.

When you have a brain injury, you don't always know what skills or memories or aptitudes you've lost until you need to call upon them and they aren't there. That's the part of brain injuries that many people know about. What may be less known is that you also gain things you never had before. You don't know what you've gained until something happens—some wonderful or necessary moment—and you discover an entirely new gift.

I found one of my new gifts when flying back to Vermont from Miami reading a newspaper about a girl in a coma with a traumatic head injury. The disconnected me was gone. There was no time to waste. I was struck with purpose like a bolt of lightning. I immediately took a taxi to the hospital.

I asked the nurses about this girl, who happened to be the same age I was when I'd had my life-changing accident. "Can I see her family?" I asked. Her family and friends were all in the waiting room — ten to fifteen people at least — and I introduced myself and told my story. I was like their daughter once. I was pronounced dead at the scene of an accident but at the last moment the paramedics found a slow faint heartbeat. I lost part of my brain and remained in a coma for months. The doctors didn't expect me to survive, never mind thrive.

They looked at me standing there, the newspaper in my hand. I could speak clearly and well. I cared about them. I was fit, and most signs of the devastating accident had been visually erased. I couldn't promise them miracles, but I could show them they are possible. I could show them that they didn't have to fall into having no hope. You have to have hope or you have little else.

The girl's mother cried and held onto me. She called me an angel from God, but I was just me — but a me with a new awareness and connection to that power that I'd never realized I had before. I wasn't just Pete Daigle. I was part of humanity and all living things and realized I had an inspirational message that could help people. By sharing it, I could make a difference.

There are two major reasons to work hard at rehabilitation, and neither of them is to become the person you were before. First, there is the need to rebuild your brain as best you can and to find ways to cope with what you've lost. The second reason is to discover the person you are now and to create the environment for new thoughts, feelings and abilities to gather and grow — because there are good things inside you waiting to be discovered like some kind of treasure hunt prizes.

I found out later that the girl in the hospital came out of her coma and was doing well. I haven't contacted her or her family since, but I wonder sometimes what she's discovered and gained. I hope her journey has been as rewarding as mine.

~Pete Daigle

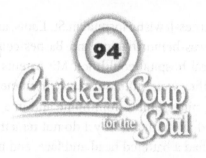

94

Good Samaritans

*We cannot pass our guardian angel's bounds, resigned or sullen,
he will hear our sighs.*

~Saint Augustine

O n May 11, 2011, I was a solo lawyer in rural Missouri, divorced and living far away from my parents and siblings. I had no children, and most of my friends lived in other cities. My local friends were married and busy with their husbands or kids most of the time. I had just experienced a bad breakup with my boyfriend, and I was not looking forward to another Friday evening alone.

My office at that time was in an historic register brick building owned by my parents. There were apartments on the floor above the office, and a back stairway connecting the office storeroom to the apartments. I remember those stairs well. They were steep, went straight up without a landing or turn, and were made of unfinished wood.

I went to the second floor that night to inspect an apartment at the request of some tenants who were moving out. On the way back to the office, I fell headlong down half a flight of stairs. I tried to break the fall with my right hand, but my wrist broke and I was knocked unconscious when my head hit the stairs.

A tenant found me and called an ambulance. Someone else found my cell phone and called my parents, who lived in Indiana. The ambulance took me to the local hospital, but I was eventually transported to Barnes-Jewish Hospital in St. Louis, an hour and a half away. My brain was hemorrhaging and Barnes could provide treatment that the local hospital could not. My parents were told about the transfer, but they were still hours away from me.

There I was, ninety miles from home and in a hospital without anyone who cared about me nearby. I do not remember it now, but I was conscious, I had a battered head and face, and my wrist was in a cast. I was probably medicated and in a great deal of pain.

Just after I was brought to my room, a man appeared by my bedside. I do not know anything about him. I do not remember if he said anything, what he looked like, or how he happened to find out about the accident. All I know is that the nurse told my parents he stayed by my bedside for hours, until just before my parents arrived in the room. The nurse assumed he was a family member because of his look of concern and the length of time that he stayed with me. He disappeared before my parents saw him.

He has not contacted me since, and I have often wondered who he was. I lived in the St. Louis area many years ago. I went to law school there, worked for a judge, and then a law firm for four years. The judge had passed away, and I had lost touch with the other people I knew in that area. There remained only a few extraordinarily kind men who were close enough to me to have stayed in that hospital room so long: a friend from school, the law school dean, an old boyfriend, and a former boss. What did not make sense, though, is that any one of those men would have stayed to see my parents. The mystery man did not. He had to have been a stranger.

My parents took over after he left. The hemorrhaging stopped and I was allowed to leave the hospital, but I was in no shape to return home and go back to work alone. My parents drove me back and forth from my home and office to their home for months, but I do not remember it.

I already had health problems that affected my ability to work before the accident. Afterward, I continued to practice law and attempted to support myself working part-time for over a year, not realizing the extent to which my intellectual skills had diminished because of the brain injury. I gradually began to understand my limitations, and closed the firm in June 2012. I moved in with my parents and applied for disability.

My parents provided my housing, but I continued getting government and charitable assistance as well as working part-time, as my health allowed, thanks to understanding supervisors, while I waited to hear on the disability claim.

I have been continually surprised that individual volunteers have appeared in my life to help just when I needed them. Strangers called the ambulance when they found me on the stairs. An anonymous person generously paid for my book in a brain injury class when I could not afford it. An assistant at the veterinarian's office let me put some pills for my dog on credit when I did not have the money for them. Two sweet women conspired to get me a paid writing assignment. And, amazingly, my mysterious guardian angel looked after me in the hospital when my family could not.

I cannot count the kindnesses extended to me for no reason except my need for help. I am grateful for all those thoughtful acts.

Most importantly, however, I am grateful that I have been taught that none of us is ever alone.

~Shelley L. Woodward

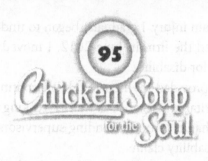

95

Soul Soup Found at Brooks Clubhouse

Wishing to be friends is quick work, but friendship is a slow ripening fruit.

~Aristotle

I opened the front door at the Brooks Clubhouse, and there stood six-foot-plus Jacob. He looked at my face and said, "I know you, but I don't know your name." Jacob is one of the last patients I worked with at the neuro-rehabilitation day treatment program before I retired. Jacob's memory wasn't bad for not having seen me for six weeks.

The room was busy with new arrivals at the front desk, some already attending to their jobs, several people on computers, others visiting and drinking coffee. Most began to gravitate to the dining room where the day begins with a community meeting around 9:30. Mona was facilitating today. The meeting moved along, bouncing from topic to topic.

"Who left the musical turtle in my chair? Let's keep it in the bathroom!"

Chappy pushes a wash bucket between the tables.

"This is my first day. I have a bad memory but I remember faces. Don't worry I'll help you with that. I sat home a long time and then I found this place. Now, I come here every day. I couldn't remember names all my life; now I can blame my brain injury. I like chocolate.

I yawn a lot, but you're not boring—I just do it. This will change your life!"

Sometimes statements were prefaced with a name, but the important thing was the message, not the name.

Kathy arrived with the Friday doughnuts—the meeting was over—time to go to work, but not until after the doughnuts!

The planning meeting for maintenance group that day included three people using wheelchairs, and jobs were open for bid. Nancy, dubbed the "disinfectant diva," would clean the light switches, Joy the sinks, and, since no one wanted the toilets, Mona volunteered to be "captain of the commodes" for the day. Off they went—Mona leading the wheelchair chain, toilet bowl brush in hand. As the group finished the first bathroom, Mike came out of the next bathroom saying "Don't go in there, seriously, don't go in there!"

Each person worked at their own job, at their own speed—there was no pressure to hurry. Rather the atmosphere was peppered with stories about smoking cigarettes, not smoking cigarettes, and lots of jokes... but always heard among the ranks were thank you, please and great job today!

It is often difficult to see the difference between the staff, volunteers and members—everyone is working to maintain the clubhouse—it's a collaboration.

This is a clubhouse run by the members. The price for membership? Brain injury. All are treated, first, as people, with strengths and weaknesses, not as impaired survivors. I observed a different kind of friendship at the clubhouse. It was touched with respect, and, sometimes, brutal honesty. Impairments were a fact of life. They were not the focus; rather solutions were the focus, searched for by all. I saw people who struggle with aphasia and hearing impairments communicate with each other—sometimes it was a hug, sometimes it was a wrestling hold—but delivered with love between cohorts.

It is a member-driven and -supported program. There are no agreements, contracts, schedules or rules intended to enforce participation. Members attend as many days as they like, and they choose what they want to work on.

I never heard, "that's not appropriate," as you hear, often, in structured rehabilitation programs, but I did hear, "that hurts my feelings," "your breath stinks," or "I feel bad when you say that."

The kitchen is abuzz with lunch prep led by Mike. Mike is one of five employees at the clubhouse. He is a TBI survivor who has dedicated his life to helping others who find themselves in the same boat. When he completed rehab, he remained connected to Brooks by volunteering to cook at the day treatment program, and when the clubhouse opened he was hired to provide leadership in the kitchen. Today it's individual pizzas, green salad and fruit, followed by Mike's birthday cake. Many need assistance to get their food onto their plates and to the table. It happens without ado, and soon everyone is happily munching on birthday cake. One of the members is a former produce man, and Mike goes with him to the farmer's market on Mondays, and they stock up on fresh fruits and vegetables for the week.

Following lunch, *Uno* is the game of choice in the main room. Members come and go, playing a few hands or staying for the entire activity. "Don't tell me what card to play, I know what I'm doing." Some can hold the cards, some use cardholders, and some have their cards on the table. Turns can take only seconds or much longer. Another game was *Would You Rather?*, a game that gives two equally silly options, and you pick one. What a hoot everyone has with this.

Many of the individuals I see, I have followed since discharge from acute inpatient rehabilitation. Some would not be able to return to competitive employment; some are not ready now. Families and friends resumed their lives, and these patients were left to sit at home all day with nowhere to go. Now they have a place to go where they are accepted, loved and guided to a fuller life... and they love it.

Ms. Alice, the matriarch of the clubhouse, completed the day treatment program and was still unable to communicate effectively. She goes to the clubhouse five days a week as she has done for the five years it has been open, and she now works in the culinary unit, leads an exercise group (when she feels like it) and readily interacts with everyone. She is, in fact, the one who had a wrestling hold on another member in the kitchen—she was giving some tough love to Don!

The Brooks Clubhouse has always been a vision of my friend Kathy and she has been able to see her dream come true. It has changed the lives of neurologically impaired individuals over the last five years. It's a haven for people who might have filled their days with television, overeating, drinking, drugs, depression, or isolation. Now there's a place to go every day. A place that offers hope, compassion, camaraderie, and a darn good time!

I retired from neuro-rehabilitation with the knowledge that individuals who suffer life-changing neurological trauma have a life-long option in Jacksonville that enables them to participate in a fuller life that they can captain.

I salute those who have supported and funded the clubhouse and Kathy, for pursuing her dream. But most off all, I salute the members for making Brooks Clubhouse their very own and very unique rehabilitation.

~Diane Kleinschmidt

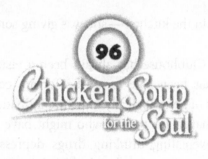

96

Giving Voice to TBI

My home is in Heaven. I'm just traveling through this world.
~Billy Graham

Whenever I think of traumatic brain injury, I listen to a recording of my first husband, Dale, singing. Having grown up singing in his father's Baptist church, Dale's baritone voice rose above most singers. His voice was powerful, yet also buttery soft. People compared him to Glen Campbell, the reigning crooner of the late 1960s. When I met Dale in a private high-school singing group, everyone knew he was destined for greatness.

I was a vocalist too, in a family of musicians. My grandmother had been a music teacher for forty years. But I had no designs on becoming a star. My soprano voice was nice enough, but I wasn't much of a soloist. Why would I need to take center stage while a talent like Dale was around? I was content to sing harmonies for songs like the Fifth Dimension's "Up, Up and Away" or sing backup for Dale's powerful vocals and solid guitar work.

Besides, my first goal was to date this heartthrob! With a shock of golden hair falling across his eyes, his easy smile lit up my teenage heart. It wasn't long before we were a couple. We dated, but I was most content when we sang together, whether sharing the stage with the likes of stars like Trini Lopez and Robert McRae or just making nursing home folks happy with our songs.

Being young and in love, we married after high school. But performing music together wasn't enough to hold our marriage together, even after he got a job as a telephone worker—just like Jimmy Webb's famous "Wichita Lineman" song. After three rocky years, we parted and went our separate ways.

Life happened and we both remarried. Years passed and I seldom even thought of those heady days when Dale and I thought he'd be a famous singing sensation. But on New Year's Eve in 1993, I dreamed of my former husband. In the dream he told me, "We should have just been friends, not spouses," and for me not to worry. "I'll be all right," he said. The dream seemed so real that it stuck with me. What did it mean?

Several weeks later, Dale's mom phoned me. A year or so earlier, she said, Dale had suffered a traumatic brain injury. He'd moved to Nashville Tennessee, to "make it" as a singer, and during a storm, a strong wind had knocked a telephone cable across the road. Dale had the lineman experience, so he attempted to move the cable to the side of the road. But it whipped around, slammed into him and he fell head first onto a concrete slab.

He survived, but barely. He had to relearn all sorts of basic things such as writing and reading. But the most tragic aspect of his TBI was that he lost his ability to sing. The day his mother phoned me, it was to say he'd passed away of an accidental drug interaction, just as he was beginning to put his life—and his music—back together. Dale's mom sounded heartbroken. "He was just starting to get back the things he'd lost," she said. "He was starting to remember how to sing again."

I wasn't a family member any longer, but I was so overcome, I couldn't speak. I still admired my ex's voice and his resolve to "go for it" in the Nashville country music scene. I asked, "When exactly did this happen?"

She paused a moment, and I thought I heard a soft whimper. "New Year's," she said. "They found him on New Year's Day."

I remembered my dream, and although it could have been coincidental, I believe he was trying to comfort me. My former mother-in-law agreed and asked for my mailing address. "There's something he would have wanted you to have," she added before we said goodbye.

For a time, I was angry that traumatic brain injury had cruelly shortened this man's life. He was too gifted, too dedicated to his art. But then I remembered my grandmother's major stroke, suffered after she'd retired from teaching music. The stroke took away her ability to speak. Yet when she needed to communicate, she could still sing. The sound of her singing without words spoke volumes about her love for me. Perhaps some good would come out of Dale's tragedy too.

A few days after Dale's mom called, a small package arrived. Inside was a professional demo recording Dale had made in Nashville before TBI robbed his voice. I rushed to play it and there was that beautiful soaring baritone, belting out a country song. I sang along and smiled — TBI stole his voice but not his spirit.

~Linda S. Clare

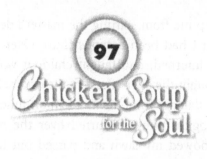

97

Once a Teacher...

*We don't receive wisdom; we discover it for ourselves after a journey
that no one can take for us or spare us.*
~Marcel Proust

One second I sat in a solid line of traffic on Interstate 70 near Broncos Stadium in Denver, Colorado. The next, my upper body pitched forward after a thunderous crash and jolt. A standard lap belt grabbed at my hips. The back of the plush captain's chair broke off behind me in the middle of the van. A hot semi-truck engine replaced the two back doors. The van slammed into another four-door sedan. I felt like a cowboy on a bucking bronco, with no way to brace myself between collisions. Other drivers pulled their untouched cars to the side of the road. Drivers rushed to the ditch to allow the first responders to render aid. Someone yelled, "Get everyone out of the vehicles! There are fluids all over the highway!" The smell of burning rubber and smoke made my adrenaline kick into overtime. My muddled brain registered how close my van had come to flying off the overpass. The blood in my mouth made the bile rise in my throat. I struggled to stay awake. My mother and sister forced me to talk until the EMTs arrived. I felt a huge lump forming on the back of my head.

Several hours later, the staff at University of Colorado Hospital in Denver diagnosed me with a concussion, severe bruising to my abdomen and hips, a sprained neck, and a locked jaw.

I returned to my home in Kansas a few days later. I was not about to let my TBI stop me from starting the master's degree program in special education I had been accepted into. Over the next several years, I studied, interned, and taught children with special needs. All the while, I fought the after-effects of the original traumatic brain injury and spinal damage from the accident on June 15, 1995.

Odd neurological things occurred over the next seven years. One hot day, I mowed my lawn and passed out in my back yard. A physical therapist put me on a Stairmaster for ten minutes and I blacked out. A couple of years later, I awoke unable to stand.

Late one Friday night, I found myself on an MRI table once again. I had lost feeling on the left side of my body. The radiologist asked if I could stay another hour for additional scans. At that moment, I knew the numbness was serious. My stomach roiled with questions. About 7:30 p.m. he strongly advised me to contact a neurosurgeon and neurologist on Monday morning.

On October 4, 2002, the neurologist confirmed a diagnosis of multiple sclerosis.

"Do you understand that there are treatments available, but no cure?" the doctor asked.

I wanted to scream, "No, I don't know anything about MS."

As I underwent treatments, I cried on the kitchen floor when I couldn't pour a glass of milk. I laughed when I walked out of my mules without feeling a thing. I fell, but I kept getting up, even if I had to humble myself to ask for help.

Some moments my symptoms felt insurmountable. My ambulation difficulties hadn't even been rectified when I lost my depth perception. I arose one Christmas morning without any vision in my left eye. It made slipping through a doorway a full-contact sport. Teaching taxed my body beyond human limits.

While doctors struggled to slow down the MS exacerbations, my inspiration came from a nine-year-old student.

Duncan spent the majority of his days in a wheelchair due to cerebral palsy, a fate I became all-too-acquainted with myself, since I started steroid treatments.

A team of teachers, including myself, tried to encourage him to operate a special computer to be his voice. Duncan seemed perfectly content to continue his silence and bob his head to say, "Yes" or "No".

Then I visited him at school during a short leave-of-absence. I'd heard that Duncan had withdrawn from everyone when I didn't return to school. There I sat in a wheelchair, weak, with an I.V. tube taped to the back of my left hand.

Duncan accessed the computer's voice and asked, "How are you?... Miss Reid... I miss you."

"I've really missed you, too," I replied. "Thank you so much for speaking. Great job! The teachers told me that you won't use your voice at school."

"Miss Reid... lie down... nurse's office."

"Duncan, you're correct. I'll have to leave soon, but I need you to help me. Other people don't know how funny and smart you are when you refuse to speak with your computer. I'll make you a deal. If you speak to your other teachers each day, my substitute teacher will turn on the speakerphone for you to call me at home. Would you like that?"

Duncan smiled, nodded his head, and said, "Yes... Yes... Yes."

Thus began Duncan's life with a voice. With each physical setback for me came new insights into the lives of my exceptional students. Duncan became my champion, as I became his.

I called technology specialists who taught me how to operate Duncan's voice output system. They visited my home and brought mobility devices to borrow until I walked independently. The same specialists, who trained me on assistive technologies for my students, now pulled me up from the quagmire of my new life. What were the odds?

For the next seven years, I fought to continue teaching. I'd received steroid infusions and physical therapy to recover most of my abilities. My career ended when the superintendent of schools decided I presented more of a liability than a benefit to the district.

People asked me if I would have skipped graduate school and chosen a different career path in life had I been diagnosed after the car accident. But I know I wouldn't have survived that first year after diagnosis if not for my students with multiple disabilities.

As a teacher, I never allowed students to entertain the idea of giving up. Together, we learned to adapt to the vast challenges tossed our way. I'm indebted to these children and their families forever. They reminded me what was most important in life—loving relationships.

Today, I'm content to help people in hospitals and schools by performing pet-assisted therapy with my companion dog, Zoey. When patients hear my story, they inquire about local organizations that provide assistance for their new physical challenges. I'm only too happy to oblige. Once a teacher, always a teacher.

~Leann Reid

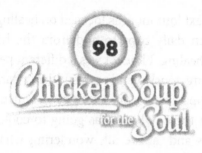

98

"Just Trauma"

*Your present circumstances don't determine where you can go;
they merely determine where you start.*

~Nido Qubein

One snowy Berkshire morning I packed up my four-wheel drive vehicle and took off on a four-hour drive. As a boarding school admissions officer, domestic and international travel was the norm for me. I don't remember anything for the next thirteen days after that morning, but my family recalls it all too well. My nine- and eleven-year-old daughters were met at the bus stop by their dad and must have known before he spoke that something was very wrong. He told them I was at a trauma center an hour away with multiple fractures as the result of a car crash on black ice.

Two weeks later, my first memory was that of an uncomfortably scratchy blanket around my neck as I was driven somewhere in an ambulance. I spent the next three weeks in a hospital near my home with daily visits from my family. I was in a cloud in which I couldn't remember names; I couldn't sleep, and all the doctors repeatedly told me that it was "just trauma." My world seemed to become one long grueling physical rehabilitation session, re-learning to walk, managing to speak with my jaws tightly wired, and trying to understand why my thinking was suddenly so strange, my memory so poor and my ability to find the right word gone.

There was no mention of brain injury.

I spent the next four months focused on healing, first with rehab at home and then daily trips to and from the hospital. However, beyond physical healing, I knew I was a different person. My balance was terrible; my previously gentle self suddenly had periods of anger or tears for no apparent reason. I fought to remember where I had to go, how to get there, what I was going to cook, how to manage household chores and, above all, wondering what had really happened to me. That began my search for the answers and battle for help.

A good patient who believed that all of my doctors certainly had my best interests at heart, I returned to work, changed employers and accepted a demanding new post. Meanwhile I read everything I could about my symptoms, and decided I had a vestibular disorder of serious concern. It made sense; my severely fractured jaw was in the same area, and so I managed to convince my case manager that I needed to have an evaluation at Massachusetts Eye and Ear Infirmary's vestibular lab.

Four years post injury, after a day of comprehensive evaluation, the result was not what I had guessed. The doctor told me it was not vestibular; rather I had sustained a severe and classic traumatic brain injury. That moment instantly changed my healing journey, and I left the office already set to begin something new—brain injury rehabilitation.

I resigned from my job and for two years I traveled across Massachusetts by train each week to meet with my neurologist, neuropsychologist, and speech therapist, as there was no brain injury rehab near my home. My homework was demanding and life changing, but I finally had the ultimate team of professionals at my side. My family planned every minute around my rehab and we all learned that it would take a lot of education and hard work for me to get to be my new best. I spent more of my days doing volunteer work for the Brain Injury Association of Massachusetts (BIA-MA) and agreed to take over the facilitation of the Berkshire Brain Injury Support Group. My life has become a fulfilling combination of rehab, volunteerism and motherhood supported by a remarkable family and new friends at the BIA-MA. I have been honored to be a member and former chair of the Massachusetts Brain Injury Advisory Board, a member of the BIA-MA board, to have sat on the board of the Brain Injury Association of America and to have worked with brain injury projects in other states.

The human spirit is resilient and brain injury tries to push each of us to our unknown limit. The struggles are many and the burdens seem intolerable, but if one can find a handful of people who are willing to learn about brain injury and link to some of the resources, other connections begin to appear. It is certainly not easy nor is it an experience any of us would choose, but each of us has skills and talents we can offer as we build a team of support. The trick is to find a sparkling glimmer of hope on the darkest of days and to stretch toward one dream at a time.

~Suzanne D.K. Doswell

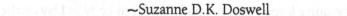

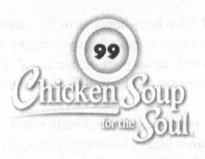

99

A Journey Back from Head Trauma

When the solution is simple, God is answering.
~Albert Einstein

The nurse leaned over my frail, bandaged body as I lay on the hospital bed. "Patti, open your mouth." My mouth remained clamped shut. I was stubborn. I was also frightened. "You have to eat to get stronger, Patti. Now please, open your mouth."

Everything the nurse said mattered. And it would have made sense to most people. Just not to me. Having survived a horrific car crash, my brain was, in many ways, starting over. I had no thoughts, no memories, no feelings, no understanding of what was normal or real or what most people know or do naturally. All I could do was respond to each moment as it happened. Yet each moment I was struggling to survive. Still, by the grace of God, there I was.

Eyewitnesses to the crash that took place on June 18, 2002 weren't sure what they saw. When the Dodge semi, going 70 mph down the highway pulling a trailer full of cars slammed into the back of the Chevy Tahoe, an off-duty registered nurse watched as what looked like a piece of laundry flew through the air. That piece of laundry was me. As the Tahoe finally came to a stop, my body plummeted back to earth. The force of the impact caused my body to slide the length of a three-story building. I lost well over sixty percent of my blood. My body was damaged beyond recognition and I fell into a coma for six weeks.

The Life Flight helicopter flew me to the nearest trauma center. After the first seventy-two hours, the doctors prepared my family. "If your daughter does wake up from her coma, she may be in a persistent vegetative state. She will never walk again or talk in complete sentences. She won't be able to see out of her right eye and she'll never be able to have any type of job or vocation."

It's hard, if not impossible, to explain what it was like waking up after suffering a traumatic brain injury. My thoughts were limited to what I could see or hear or touch. My brain was broken. I had no memory of the harrowing event that had landed me in that hospital bed. I certainly didn't realize then that nothing in my life would ever be the same again. As I lay in that bed at Baylor Institute for Rehabilitation in Dallas, my brain and body had only just begun their slow crawl back to life and health.

I don't remember much, if anything, of my time coming out of the coma. The days are a blur. The visits from friends and family and the care I received from so many nurses and doctors during my recovery are all stories I have been told. For me, that time is and probably always will be a complete blank.

Memories of my life are like snapshots in a photo album that someone explained to me. I couldn't comprehend the words people were saying, but I could recognize their nonverbal communication. That's what I paid attention to the most—the inflection in my dad's voice, the eye contact between my mother and me, my brother's habit of holding my hand, a hug from a friend. This was the language that spoke volumes to me, the only language I knew.

Re-learning life following traumatic brain injury requires more than one try. Step by step, we learn to live again. Functioning in the real world demands attention and remembrance. These two traits are extremely difficult for a recovering head trauma survivor. Even as you're learning new things, you discover that a lot of information can enter your brain and quickly skip right back out. Things come and go so quickly.

The long, day-by-day process of recovery that started in 2002 shows no sign of ending. I still easily forget things on a daily basis. It's hard work and sometimes I get frustrated. What I once could do so easily and so enjoyably now demands a substantial amount of my mental energy. Before the crash, I was a good listener, a counselor-type of person. Now, as I cope with the deficits, I still like listening to and helping others, but I simply don't have as much "brain fuel" as I used to have.

I have learned that there's an upside to short-term memory loss. First of all, I forget many of the mean, hurtful things people say and do. My memory storage bank doesn't hold much for long. A lot of it disappears, especially the details. By the same token, when I hear good news or read something positive, whether it's the second, third, or forty-eighth time, I will celebrate as if I'm hearing it for the first time. It's all new and fresh to me!

I wonder today if I could have made it through the struggles of my ordeal so well if it weren't for the testimony of Holocaust survivor and author, Corrie Ten Boom. My Aunt Jenny introduced me to her books, though I doubt she realized the impact this amazing woman's story would have on my life. Corrie's tale of steadfast faith in the face of adversity gripped my heart and my imagination. How could she not only endure such evil, but come through it with such a deep and abiding belief in God's love? God used the strength of this courageous Dutch woman to prepare me for the adversity I would face in my own life as a traumatic brain injury survivor. Her strength in dealing with loss stayed with me. And her steadfast faith in the goodness of God helped give me the courage I needed to cope.

What I've gone through since the crash has presented me with many unexpected opportunities to give back, to give something that I've learned in order to help others with the knowledge I've gained along this journey, very much like the apostle Paul teaches us in 2 Cor. 1:3,4. Yes, life is hard, but God is good.

So, as long as God gives me breath and strength and a voice, I will continue to use this gift of life to live my motto: "Make a Difference Now!" I will not squander these blessings but share them. After all, everything I have belongs to God. I am not my own. I am His. He has had a purpose and a plan for all that has happened to me from the moment I hopped in that SUV and headed toward Tyler, Texas.

God has a purpose for you too. I pray you find it… and use it to make the kind of difference only you can!

~Patti Foster

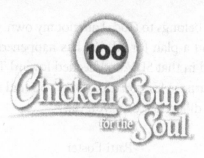

100

The Soldier Is My Side-Walker

Age merely shows what children we remain.
~Johann Wolfgang von Goethe

I knocked on the door to Dan's room. "Dan, can I come in?"

"Yeah."

I opened the door and stepped inside. It took a few moments for my eyes to find Dan. His blurry outline was hidden under the covers in the darkened room.

"Are you going to sleep all day?" I asked.

"Sure, why not?" he said flatly.

"Well for one thing, you are wasting a gorgeous day by hiding in this cave."

Piles of paper, loose change, cups, a hammer, and nails littered the top of his bureau. Piles of laundry on the floor and partially opened drawers with clothing spilling out gave the place a ransacked look.

"Yeah, well there's nothing for me to get up for."

"That isn't true."

"Oh yeah? What do I have to get up for? What do I have to do? Whatever I do doesn't mean anything. I don't do anything that has any real meaning. And nobody cares if I stay in bed all day or not."

"Dan, that's absolutely not true."

"Really, who cares?"

"I do," I replied firmly, truthfully. "I care. The rest of the staff that works here care. The other residents care. We all care."

Silence.

"Have you taken a shower yet today?"

"No."

"How about getting up, taking a shower, and then we'll talk while you have your breakfast?"

He offered a lackluster, "Okay."

I considered that he might have acquiesced in order to get rid of me, but preferred to think that some of what I do makes a difference. Getting him up was just the beginning.

While Dan was taking his shower, I tried to figure out what I could say to him that would help him find a reason to care about his life. Dan is a tall, muscular, attractive young man who sustained a serious traumatic brain injury while he was serving in the United States Army. His TBI was so severe that he wasn't expected to live. His rehabilitation has taken over two years and will go on for as long as Dan continues to show improvement in his struggles with memory problems, mood swings, headaches, chronic pain, and insomnia.

When I first met Dan, I was impressed with his intelligence and his motivation to get on with his life. He had been selected to participate in a new all-military transitional house located in Germantown, Maryland for continued rehabilitation and transition back to civilian life. I had been hired as the occupational therapist to work with the soldiers and veterans there. Dan's brain injury affected his mood and his mood greatly affected his behavior. This became the focal point of our work together.

Forty-five minutes later, Dan stood before me, freshly showered and ready to face the day. Standing up, he began to eat his breakfast near the sink.

"Why don't you sit down and eat your breakfast at the table so we can talk?"

He moved to the table and looked down into his cereal, listening as he ate.

"I know that you're depressed, that you're in pain, and that you don't want to be here. I understand that you feel trapped and lost. I'd like to help you to move forward."

"What do you mean?"

"As an occupational therapist, I help people find a way to do the things they value. What kinds of things do you like to do?"

"I like to play the guitar. I like to build things."

"And what would you like to do if you could do anything?" I continued.

"Well, what I'd really like to do is work with kids. They don't expect a lot from you and they're fun to be around."

I thought for a few minutes and then an idea came to me.

"Would you be willing to volunteer some of your time?"

"Sure. I've got nothing but time these days."

"In addition to working here, I work at a therapeutic riding center with kids who have neurological and developmental disorders."

"What do you do there?"

"I work as an occupational therapist, but I do a form of OT called hippotherapy."

"What's that?"

I could almost see the wheels turning in his head and imagined him picturing hippopotamuses.

"Hippo, in Greek, means horse. The children receive their therapy on horseback."

"How exactly does that work?"

"We work as a team. There's a leader who leads the horse, myself the therapist, the patient or child on the horse, and a side-walker. I think you'd be great as a side-walker."

Dan's expression told me that he was considering my idea.

"Why don't you come to the riding center next week? If you like what you see, you can fill out the volunteer application. Once you complete the short training, you will be an official side-walker."

And so, Dan joined my team. He was self-conscious about not being able to remember everyone's names, but I assured him that he could ask people for their names as often as he needed to. This was truly a forgiving environment.

The first time Dan served as my side-walker, I realized what a treasure he was. Not only was he tall and strong, but he interacted with the kids without my having to tell him what to do. He smiled and sang, encouraged and reassured. I had worked with adults throughout most of my career and envied his easy way with the children. Dan was a natural.

Once our sessions were over for the day, Dan asked "What's wrong with them?"

I told him about each child and why they needed occupational therapy and how using the horse helped them to sense what normal movement feels like. I stressed that each child had a unique set of needs.

Dan said, "I feel lucky compared to them."

"Me, too. Some days when things look dark, I think of these kids. They remind me that I have a lot to be thankful for."

From then on, whenever I worked at the riding center and Dan was volunteering, I insisted on having him as my side-walker. I trusted his judgment. I frequently shared with him my confidence in his skills. He pointed out improvements in the children we worked with and expressed pride at being an integral part of their therapy.

"When I'm at the center, I feel good about what I'm doing. I feel my best when I'm there and when I'm doing something useful. It just makes me feel good."

Dan has made an important contribution to the children we work with. They look for him and ask for him. Some of them run up to him and wrap their arms around him in greeting. Their parents are impressed with both Dan and his story. They have great respect for his military service, for having survived a traumatic brain injury, and for having the devotion to help others whose needs are greater than his.

~Amy Soscia

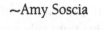

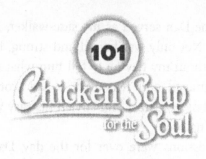

The Gift

God gave us the gift of life; it is up to us to give ourselves the gift of living well.

~Voltaire

I
n the quiet of the car, I studied his profile. My teenage son had the promise of manhood shining in his face while, if I looked carefully enough, I could still see the last flickers of the beautiful child Matthew once was. His father, Steven, had wept silent tears the night before as we watched that face under the cold compress covering his eyes. The headache had been especially brutal. Even with the lights out, the room silent, and the damp cloth in place, we'd watched as our child soundlessly writhed on the bed.

And the guilt was just too much.

Steven "knew" it wasn't his fault. He'd been told so a thousand times. But, his son had fallen on his watch. Literally. Steven had turned from the phone just in time to look in horror as his baby reached out to wave to him from the second story landing... and fell head first onto the stair below. The impact shattered his skull as the thirteen-month-old began to scream out the agony of his injury.

Across town at the time, I'd been called to come and say goodbye to my baby, as he appeared to be losing his fight for life in the hospital. When he began to improve, we'd been warned that he would never walk or talk or use his right side.

And, yet, he did. Matthew's life has been a series of little miracles. He survived two incredibly difficult, experimental, brain surgeries.

He learned to walk. He stopped dragging his right side and began to do the impossible. He ran. He laughed. He talked up a storm.

But life was also hard. Too much reading or writing or thinking and he'd be struck by major migraines. At that moment, he'd lose all ability to tolerate print... or even, light. And, he was often stricken every day.

At four, he ran away from preschool and headed home with his scissors. He was so embarrassed that he couldn't cut when all the other kids could that he stole the supplies and brought them home so I could teach him. And we tried. And tried. But, despite all our efforts for all those years, he would be in seventh grade before he'd really get the hang of scissors.

He'd learned to read in kindergarten, then lost the letter "F" in second grade. He forgot how to write it, or say it, or decode it. And so it went.

Testing for learning disabilities, we discovered a seizure disorder that clocked as many as two hundred seizures in twenty minutes. Because the emotional centers of his brain were also destroyed, Matthew suffered from terrible anxiety. Night terrors would send him racing around the house, tearing away from some unseen danger. For years he slept between his sisters. And, when one particularly insensitive teacher yelled at him, my son threw a blanket over his head and slammed his body into the wall for an hour.

And yet, here he sat next to me, confident, competent and caring. Each small miracle feeding into the next until here he was; he could have been any teen on the edge of adulthood.

"How are you?" I asked

"Fine. Why?" he replied.

"That was a pretty awful headache last night."

"Yeah, it was."

"Your dad was feeling really bad that you had to suffer like that."

"What do you mean?" asked my son, turning to me in utter surprise.

"Well, you know, sometimes he feels very guilty for letting you fall. Last night was a bad one for him, too."

"You're kidding." Matt was incredulous. Steven's shame over Matt's accident made "the blame" a topic that was seldom discussed.

"No, I'm not. Your dad really suffers about your injury."

"But, Mom," began my boy. "I like my brain injury."

"What?" I wasn't sure I'd heard him correctly.

"Well, yeah," he said. "You know, I'm really smart. I know I'm smart. But, if I were just smart, I could turn into a real arrogant jerk thinking everything was easy and I deserved it to be easy. But, instead, I struggle because of my brain injury. I can be really smart on one hand, but then things can be incredibly hard on the other." Then Matthew flashed that smile that told me the punch line was coming. "My brain injury keeps me humble about my magnificence!" He stopped for a moment and thought, before quietly adding, "It's a gift." That night, Matthew sat down with his dad and told him what he'd told me and I watched as Steven collapsed into his son's embrace.

Today, Matt is a teacher. He works with severely autistic and developmentally disabled young men. He takes on the most difficult students at school because, as he says, he really understands their struggles and somehow, instinctively, knows how to get through to them and help them reach their full potential. My son, too, has reached his full potential: so much more than I'd feared on that fateful day in the hospital—yet, even more than I'd dreamed on the day he was born. He's found his calling—a calling that embraces both his "smartness" and his disability as real attributes. And, "his boys" are the recipients of both.

He says it's his gift.

~Susan Traugh

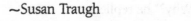

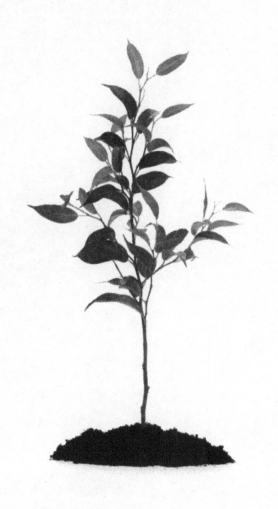

Recovering *from* Traumatic Brain Injuries

Meet Our Contributors

Meet Our Authors

About Lee Woodruff
and the Bob Woodruff Foundation

Thank You

About Chicken Soup for the Soul

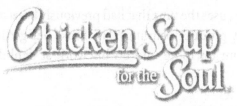

Meet Our Contributors

Richard E. Berg is an artist and advocate. He co-hosts two poetry venues in southeastern Massachusetts and competes at poetry slams in Providence and Boston. His first poetry book is due out in fall 2014. Richard speaks to organizations about the effects of brain injury on survivors and families. He is a multiple trauma and brain injury survivor.

Bonnie L. Beuth received her Bachelor of Science degree, *summa cum laude*, in Information Systems and works in the learning and development field. She is a founding member of the Legal Technology Core Competencies Certification Coalition and has many pastimes, including writing and keeping up with a large group of friends.

Jon Blair has a fantastic sense of humor and can find humor in everything. He believes that humor has gotten him through a lot of his ordeal and believes having faith and humor can't go wrong. He would like to thank Paula Schmidt and the Brain Injury Association for their support in writing this story.

Christine Blue has a Bachelor of Science degree in Music Education and her Master of Arts degree from CWRU. She teaches music and band in Mentor, OH, and speaks at TBI conferences about the use of music therapy as an aid in recovery. She loves her husband and daughter and enjoys reading, traveling, and listening to live music.

Dan Bornstein, who has worked for the family business in Portland,

ME since 2008, uses the time that had previously been used to produce writing to now produce paintings. He thinks he's getting pretty good too. E-mail him for more info on his work at danbdoodles@gmail.com.

Sage de Beixedon Breslin, Ph.D is a Licensed Psychologist and Intuitive Consultant. She is an accomplished author and screenwriter, generating material to inspire and touch those who have struggled with life's challenges. Her books, stories, and chapters are available on her website at www.HealingHeartCenter.org.

Sandra L. Brown lives on the prairies of Saskatchewan. She has two married sons and three grandchildren of whom she is very proud. Sandra works full-time in the oil industry and enjoys paleontology, museums, hockey and writing. Her advice to anyone recovering from a head injury is to "enjoy the miracle of each new day!"

Kelly Buttiglieri received her B.A. degree with honors from Boston College in 1989 and J.D. degree with honors from Suffolk University Law School in 1994. She is married, has a fourteen-year-old son and nine-year-old daughter. Kelly has worked for the Brain Injury Association of Massachusetts for eight years. She enjoys reading and gardening.

Michele Camacho, e-mail and campaign copywriter, helps results-oriented entrepreneurs get the most from every e-mail with messages that engage, enlighten as well as create stories that keeps prospects engaged. Learn more at www.MicheleCamacho.com.

Joseph Caminiti has worked for Turtle & Hughes for twenty-five years. He enjoys graphic and media design, photography, and writing. Joseph volunteers for the Brain Injury Alliance of New Jersey and is a member of the Council for Head Injured Community, helping lobby for laws that help people with brain injuries live better lives.

Marshall Campbell was ordained to the ministry at the Historic Little Rock Missionary Baptist Church by Rev. Dr. Jim Holley in 1999. He took journalism in high school and wrote a column for the school paper. He is married with three girls. Marshall enjoys golfing, bowling and has finished his novel, a biography, *Living While Black In America*.

Betty B. Cantwell received her B.A. degree from University of Texas at Arlington and her MFA degree from Texas Woman's University. Her writings have been published in Guideposts books and *Christian Woman* magazine. She enjoys poetry and writing for young children. She lives with her husband Don in Arlington, TX.

Paul Ceretto lives in Wisconsin with his two birds, Sonny and Boo Boo. He operates paulceretto.com, and is dedicated to furthering his writing career and the integrity of the written word. In his second life for five and half years now, he feels five. A statement for those who know him is all too true.

Barbara Chandler is a writer, teacher, public speaking coach and non-profit fundraiser. She earned her master's degree in speech communication from the University of Nebraska at Omaha.

Linda S. Clare is a multi-published, award-winning author of nonfiction and fiction. Her most recent release is *A Sky Without Stars* from Abingdon Press (2014). She lives in Eugene, OR with her husband, four grown children, two grandsons and three wayward cats.

Kim Conrad is a powerful spirit. Clients have said, "Kim Conrad is a gift! Her ability is extraordinary." She combines her master's in psychology, theatrical background, acute intuition, training as a Reiki Master, along with her workshops and "word-smithing" to inspire freedom at every turn. Learn more at www.KimConrad.com.

Kirsten Corrigan received her B.A. degree from Luther College and her M.A. degree from The University of Iowa. She retired from a career in finance to focus on being Mom to her son, Ryan. Kirsten enjoys photography, running, teaching aqua aerobics, writing, and educating others about shaken baby. E-mail her at kirsten.r.corrigan@ gmail.com.

Melissa Cronin holds a B.S. degree in Nursing from Boston University and an MFA degree in Creative Nonfiction from Vermont College of Fine Arts. She lives with her husband, John, in South Burlington, VT. She is working on a memoir and writes for a local newspaper. Melissa enjoys playing the Irish fiddle and riding her bicycle.

Pete Daigle is a TBI survivor who has spent much of his life since his initial recovery (i.e. ER, ICU, hospital rehab) obtaining the best life skills to enable himself, and anyone with a TBI, to live well! He is also a board member of the Brain Injury Association of Vermont and is very proactive in their support.

Holly Daubenspeck received her Bachelor of Arts degree in Music, with honors, in 2012. Since then, she has undergone intensive speech, physical, occupational and other therapies as part of her healing process post-accident. She would like to complete student teaching one day and then attend grad school — perhaps in music therapy.

Stephanie Davenport is a freelance writer, mom and yoga enthusiast in central Illinois. These days she's passionate about healthy living, her two kids and a great cup of coffee.

Prior to sustaining a TBI in 2004, **Jen de Jong** was a marketing director for a publishing company and wrote her first book, *Generation Ex*. Since her TBI, Jen has taken up quilting and blogging at deJongDreamHouse.com. She lives with her husband and son in Ohio.

Suzanne D.K. Doswell received her Bachelor of Arts degree from the Western College in 1974. She and her husband live in the Berkshires and have two inspiring daughters and creative grandchildren. Suzanne continues her professional work in the brain injury field and teaches visual arts to artists with disabilities.

Murray Dunlap's work has appeared in approximately fifty magazines and journals. His stories have been nominated for the Pushcart Prize three times, as well as to Best New American Voices once, and his first book—an early draft of *Bastard Blue* (then called *Alabama*)—was a finalist for the Maurice Prize in Fiction.

Dr. Christine Y. Durham, author of *Unlocking My Brain; Through the Labyrinth of Acquired Brain Injury*, shares her story of how she regained her life after brain injury to inspire others to make the best of brain injury. Christine is Victorian Senior Australian of the Year 2014 and one of BrainLink's Women of Achievement.

Anita Dziwura received her Ph.D in Economics from Fordham University in 1990. She has three sons and lives with them and her husband, Joe, in Westchester, NY. Anita enjoys skiing, playing the violin, attending concerts, and playing hockey with her sons.

Joy Engelsman received her Bachelor of Arts degree from Calvin College and earned a Master's of Divinity degree from Denver Seminary. She has travelled extensively, including a 'round-the-world trip with her husband and two daughters. Joy writes, speaks, coaches speakers and serves as a creativity consultant.

Jane Allen Farmer is a park ranger with the National Park Service. She works in the Interpretation and Education Division. In her free time, she visits with her two therapy dogs, plays with her two non-therapy dogs and three cats, and enjoys riding her horses.

Donna Fitzpatrick received her Associate of Arts Degree, with honors, in Journalism/Communication in 2013 from Sussex County Community College in New Jersey, graduating Phi Theta Kappa. She enjoys photography. Donna would like to dedicate this story to her family, friends and Doris T., who provided unconditional love and support.

For over a decade, **Patti Foster** was a radio host in Christian broadcasting. Today, she travels and shares her TBI story in the hope it will inspire others. In 2013, Patti released her biography, *Coping with Traumatic Brain Injury: One Woman's Journey from Death to Life.* Patti lives her motto: M.A.D. Now! (Make a Difference Now!)

Vanessa Friedrich is a professional equestrian and native German. After recovering from a severe horse riding accident she became a therapeutic riding instructor and now teaches horsemanship skills to people with disabilities. She started her writing career with her own story about recovery. Vanessa currently lives in South Carolina.

Melissa A. Gertz received her Juris Doctor degree in 2005 from Rutgers School of Law-Newark. This year marks the tenth anniversary of her TBI, and the fifth anniversary of the non-profit, the Community Justice Center. When not working, you can find Melissa exploring new beaches and microbreweries, and of course, working with Basset Hounds.

Arlene Rains Graber is an award-winning journalist, novelist, and devotional writer in Wichita, KS. She is the author of four books. *The Cape Elizabeth Ocean Avenue Society* is the second novel in the Plane Tree series, and is available on Amazon.com. Visit her at arlenerainsgraber.com.

Carolyn Graham is a wife, mother and grandmother. She has lived in Texas her entire life. She enjoys reading, writing and "not" arithmetic. She has been published in *Guideposts*, *Angels on Earth* and *Mysterious*

Ways magazines. She spends her free time writing and hopes to one day publish a children's book.

David A. Grant is a writer based in New Hampshire and the author of *Metamorphosis, Surviving Brain Injury*. David is also a contributing writer to *Brain Injury Journey* magazine. A survivor of a harrowing cycling accident in 2010, David openly shares his experience, strength and hope as a brain injury survivor.

Marian Green received her degree in biblical studies from Indiana Wesleyan University. Marian loves empowering women through their understanding of scripture and teaches at women's events across the country. Connect with her at uprootedandundone.wordpress.com.

Annette Gulati is a freelance writer living with her family in Portland, OR. She has published more than seventy-five stories, articles, essays, poems, and activities in numerous magazines and newspapers. Visit her at www.annettegulati.com.

Pattie Welek Hall is the author of a completed memoir, *A Mother's Dance*, based on her son's traumatic brain injury. She lives in Charleston, SC, where she hosts Joy Radio, a monthly Internet talk show with interviews of nationally renowned authors. Pattie is the mother of three grown children who are the loves of her life.

Maryanne Higley Hamilton received her BSEd-Art degree from Florida International University, and a Masters of Art Therapy degree from Vermont College. A published author, she is an art therapist at Leepa-Rattner Museum of Art. She enjoys traveling, creating art, writing children's books, and playing her clarinet in a large marching band.

Jan Heinitz is a single mother of two girls. She teaches counseling skills at a private university; many of her students are teachers who work with children who are at-risk. Jan was inspired to write about her daughter Christina's accident and how the accident affected her family's life.

Justine Johnston Hemmestad is a wife, mother of seven children (ages 5-21), and a writer for over twenty years. Currently she's also enrolled in the BLS program at The University of Iowa and has taken several Iowa Writers' Workshop, Poetry, and Playwrights Workshop courses, with a goal of one day teaching writing.

Kristen Hyde has a degree in marketing, worked as a wedding/portrait photographer, and currently has a business scanning photos and teaching photo/memory preservation. Kristen also creates photo and family storybooks, cards and other keepsakes, and has designs featured in a catalog and as templates. Learn more at lifememoriespreserved.com.

Sarah Jenkins received her Bachelor's of Science degree, with honors, and is pursuing a master's degree in forensics. With love and dedication, their family has chosen to thrive and excel. Sarah is a member of Hearts of Valor, an organization created by Operation Homefront. She hopes her story inspires others to erase the hidden wounds from this war.

Johnkle used to write a lot (all unshared) before his accident. Afterwards Johnkle could not find the motivation to do so, until this story. Johnkle listens to heavy metal, formerly volunteered at a long-term care home, and loves his cat. Johnkle hopes other people can see/find the experience in this story.

Upon graduating from Johns Hopkins University at the tender age of nineteen, **Larry C. Kerpelman** went on to earn his Ph.D in Psychology from the University of Rochester. His career has encompassed research, teaching, and writing activities in several organizations. Now retired, he spends his time writing, gardening, and walking.

Sarah Kishpaugh earned her MFA degree in Creative Writing in 2014. She works as a creative writing teacher and freelance editor and writer. Her essays have appeared in *The New York Times*, Salon.com and BrainLine.org. She is looking for a publisher for her first book, a memoir.

Diane Kleinschmidt received her B.S. and M.S. degrees from Florida State University. She recently retired after thirty-five years working in neuro rehab. She enjoys cooking, gardening, reading, and spending time with her family including two black Labs—Lola and Stringer.

Cheryl Koenig resides in Sydney, Australia. She is happily married with two inspiring sons. She is an author, motivational speaker, caregiver. She recently received the prestigious honor of the Medal of the Order of Australia—for services to people with disabilities, their families and caregivers. Learn more at www.cherylkoenig.com.

Annette Langer, third-time Chicken Soup for the Soul contributor, combines humor with storytelling. *Healing through Humor: Change Your Focus, Change Your Life!* details her triumphs from brain injury to breast cancer. *A Funny Thing Happened on My Way to the World* follows her travels to all seven continents. Visit www.AnnetteLanger.com.

Catherine LeBlanc has a Bachelor of Health Sciences and Physician's Assistant certificate from Duke University. She is a former ice hockey wing, soccer and team handball goalkeeper. Living in Cambridge, MA with her son and cat, her neuro rehab continues. She looks forward to discovering her next career.

Janna Leyde is an author and yoga teacher living in Pittsburgh, PA. Her memoir, *He Never Liked Cake*, tells the story of growing up with her father's TBI. Her second book, *Move Feel Think*, is a guidebook of twenty yoga poses specifically designed for those living with TBI and trauma.

Sandra A. Madden, a graduate of the S.I. Newhouse School of Communications at Syracuse University, is a photographer and writer, an administrative assistant at the Brain Injury Association of Massachusetts (BIA-MA), and a brain injury survivor. She is in the initial phase of publishing her first book, *Hearts All Around Us*.

Shawn Marie Mann lives in Pennsylvania. She spends her non-writing time visiting amusement parks and day tripping with her family. Her favorite color is orange. You can contact her through her website at www.shawnmariemann.com.

Bette Matero is a retired childcare professional, the mother of three grown children and grandmother of one. She worked for over thirty years to increase the quality of childcare in Colorado, where she lived most of her adult life. She and her husband, Del, live in Arizona, where she is writing her first novel.

Dee Dee McNeil is a freelance journalist, poet, singer/songwriter and educator. She has performed as a jazz singer in over twenty countries and is a Motown Records songwriter from Detroit, MI. She writes a music blog for www.lajazz.com. Her poetry book *Haiku in My Neighborhood* was published in 2012 with photographs by Roland Charles.

Anneli Norrland lives in the Rocky Mountains of Colorado.

Janine L. Osburn resides in Mendon, MA with her family.

Celeste Palmer is the founder of Bridging the Gap (www.tbibridge.org), a non-profit providing resources to help TBI survivors. She writes, speaks and provides life coaching to help others learn mindfulness and find their happiness. She has three children and two grandchildren, and enjoys golf, travel, knitting and swimming.

Elise Daly Parker is a writer, editor, blogger, writing coach. Married for thirty years, she is mom to four daughters, one son-in-law, and a new grandmother. She is co-founder of CirclesOfFaith.org. Elise believes that our stories matter and have power to inform, reform, and transform lives. E-mail her at elisedalyparker@gmail.com.

Brittany Perry lives in the mountains of West Virginia. She has been published in Chicken Soup for the Soul, attended Concord University, and the 2007 WV's Governor's School for the Arts for creative writing. She likes reviewing books on YouTube, spending time with her family, and writing. E-mail her at ilovebeingmommy91711@hotmail.com.

Cecile Proctor is a full-time student at the University of New Brunswick and the provincial contact for the Brain Injury Association of Canada. She is working towards an honors degree in psychology with a minor in cognitive neuroscience. She plans to continue her education to join the field of neuropsychology.

Tina Rapp is a writer and editor living in southwestern New Hampshire. Her work has appeared in various venues including New Hampshire Public Radio, *Yankee Magazine* books, *Concrete Wolf*, *Post* magazine, *Smoky Quartz*, and *Adanna Literary Journal*. She was an editor of *Shadow and Light—A Literary Anthology on Memory*.

Rosemary Rawlins is the author of *Learning by Accident: A Caregiver's True Story of Fear, Family and Hope*. Rosemary has written over sixty caregiving blog posts for BrainLine.org and is a frequent contributor to the magazine, *Brain Injury Journey*. She is a frequent keynote speaker and advocate for the TBI community.

Donna Reeve began writing after a car accident at sixteen left her with amnesia. Through writing, she made sense of an unknown world. She continues to write for the love and healing it brings. Watch for *Mirror, Mirror*, her memoir about overcoming her limitations to live out a normal life with her beloved husband and two sons.

Leann Reid holds a master's degree in special education and retired from teaching due to the effects of MS. She lives in Kansas City with her faithful companion dog, Zoey. They visit hundreds of people a year through the Pet Partners program. Her blog is www.ReidtheFinePrint. wordpress.com. She writes from experiences.

Forced into early retirement, **Cheryl Richards** searched for redirection and renewed passion. Writing short stories and publishing a novel based on the true events in the life of her great-grandfather, she found her passion again. She is currently working on her second novel. E-mail her at cherylrichards403@gmail.com.

Heather Roach has been teaching elementary school in Tennessee since 2001. She and Henry were married in 2002. Her story was written about five and a half years after Henry's accident in 2008 left him with a severe TBI. She hopes to encourage other caregivers of TBI survivors to rely on the Lord for guidance and to never give up.

Julie Sanderson has focused her career on helping people. She taught fifth grade before becoming a police officer. She is involved with a church camp and foster care. She now works with alcoholics on probation. Julie enjoys hiking with her dog in the woods near Lake Michigan. E-mail her at juliesanderson70@gmail.com.

Jim Scott graduated in 2006 from The University of Tampa with a B.S. degree in Economics. Jim sustained a severe TBI in a car accident on July 4, 2006. Following two years of rehab, in which he relearned daily living functions, he is trying to help others through speaking and the publishing of his memoir, *More Than a Speed Bump*.

Michael Jordan Segal is a husband, father, social worker, freelance author (including *Possible*, a CD/download of twelve stories), inspirational speaker, and works at a Level I trauma center offering emotional support. He's had many stories published in Chicken

Soup for the Soul books. To contact Mike or order his CD, visit www. InspirationByMike.com.

Richard C. Senelick, MD is a neurologist who specializes in neurorehabilitation and brain injury. He is the Medical Director of HealthSouth RIOSA (Rehabilitation Institute of San Antonio) and the Editor in Chief of HealthSouth Press. He is a regular contributor to *The Huffington Post* and *The Atlantic*.

Jennifer Sienes has a bachelor's degree in psychology and a master's degree in education. In 2007, she left teaching middle school to write full-time and has three short stories published in *Inspire Faith* anthology. She spends her days writing contemporary women's fiction and partnering in her chiropractor-husband's practice.

Sheri Siwek teaches high school English and journalism in Phoenix, AZ. Her son Richard continues his road to a successful recovery and will attend Arizona State University this fall.

Belinda Howard Smith and husband Steve reared six children in Austin, TX, and recently began a new chapter of life in the rural community of Wimberley, TX as owners of a B&B/Retreat Center. When not making beds and cooking breakfast, Belinda enjoys Bible study, crafts, scrapbooking, and writing.

Amy Soscia works as an occupational therapist with individuals who have brain injuries, mental health issues, and neurological disorders. She will graduate from Albertus Magnus College in May 2014 with an MFA in Writing. Amy is working on her first novel entitled *The Frozen Game*. E-mail her at pawsnwrite@verizon.net.

Barbara Stahura is a writer and certified journal facilitator who guides people with brain injury and family caregivers in harnessing the power of journaling for themselves. She lives in Southern Indiana with her husband, Ken Willingham, who is thriving after a traumatic brain injury in 2003, and their cat, Goldie.

When her long career as a psychiatric nurse abruptly ended with a TBI, **Helen Stewart** found meaningful work as an outreach coordinator with the Brain Injury Association of Massachusetts. She is the mother of three adventurous adult children. She was inspired to write this story after meeting Jenn Richardson at a contra dance.

Mike Strand continued working for Andersen Windows another twenty-four years after his accident before retiring to fulfill his dream of acquiring a B.A. degree in English Literature, which he earned in 2014. He is a writer and a wedding officiant. He and his wife Linda live in Oakdale, MN.

Dr. Sullivan received her medical degree from Michigan State University. She no longer practices due to the consequences of repetitive concussions. She is the author of *Brain Injury Survival Kit, 365 Tips, Tools & Tricks to Deal with Cognitive Function Loss* and does TBI/BI presentations for professionals and survivors/caregivers.

Tyler Tatasciore has since graduated from Humber College and entered the world of professional 3D art. He continues to update his work and you can see it at tylertatascore.com.

Dale Taylor earned bachelor's, master's, and doctoral degrees from The University of Kansas. He wrote and recorded a published folk song album, wrote two books, many chapters and numerous journal articles. With his wife, he enjoys sailboat racing, skiing, ballroom and swing dancing, and world travel for teaching and speaking.

Susan Traugh holds a master's degree in education and has been writing award-winning books and curricula for thirty years. She has used her experience with Matthew and her two equally amazing daughters, both of whom have disabilities, to focus her work on special needs kids. Her work can be seen at susantraugh.com.

Angela Leigh Tucker survived a car crash in 2008 that killed her young husband Rich. She sustained a traumatic brain injury, and has been growing, learning and healing ever since. She has bachelor degrees in public relations and organizational communication from the University of Central Florida.

Mary Varga is a Certified Personal Trainer and Senior Fitness Instructor. She is also the survivor of a traumatic brain injury in 1997. Mary has a business leading senior exercise classes. She is a member of Louisville Christian Writers, planning to write more inspirational stories. Her son, Andrew, is seventeen years old.

Kay Ward graduated from Worcester University in England in 1995 with a Bachelor of Arts degree in English Literature with honours. She immigrated to Perth, Western Australia with her husband and two sons in 1996, where she teaches English to overseas students. E-mail her at kward58@iinet.net.au.

Barbara J. Webster is the author of *Lost & Found: A Survivor's Guide for Reconstructing Life After a Brain Injury*, Lash & Associates Publishing. This collection of "brain injury survivor wisdom" is packed with tips, tools and strategies to assist survivors in continuing their healing and rehabilitation process.

Robin Lee Rice Whittaker received her B.S. degree in Marketing from Penn State in 1985. She has two children and currently resides in Eliot, ME. For twenty years she owned and operated a successful tourist destination in Portsmouth, NH, where she pursued and applied her love of marketing and hosting local interns.

Jennifer Wiche received several certificates and a degree from the University of the Fraser Valley from 2005 to 2010. Although she can no longer become a teacher, her life will be fulfilled with the love of her daughter Serenity and her husband Ray.

Lex Wilson is a writer and actor in Carrboro, NC.

Shelley L. Woodward graduated from law school at Washington University in St. Louis in 1986. She practiced law until June 2012, when she moved to Evansville, IN to be near family. She plans to do more writing in the future.

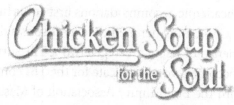

Meet Our Authors

Amy Newmark has been Chicken Soup for the Soul's publisher, coauthor, and editor-in-chief for the last six years, after a 30-year career as a writer, speaker, financial analyst, and business executive in the worlds of finance and telecommunications. Amy is a Chartered Financial Analyst and a *magna cum laude* graduate of Harvard College, where she majored in Portuguese, minored in French, and traveled extensively. She and her husband have four grown children.

After a long career writing books on telecommunications, voluminous financial reports, business plans, and corporate press releases, Chicken Soup for the Soul is a breath of fresh air for Amy. She loves creating these life-changing books for Chicken Soup for the Soul's wonderful readers. She has coauthored and/or edited more than 100 Chicken Soup for the Soul books.

You can reach Amy with any questions or comments through webmaster@chickensoupforthesoul.com and you can follow her on Twitter @amynewmark or @chickensoupsoul.

Carolyn Roy-Bornstein is a practicing pediatrician who has been treating children and their families for twenty years. After working in emergency rooms and urban health centers, on staff at Tufts University and the University of Massachusetts Medical School, she has been in private practice for the past five years.

Ten years ago, her son Neil was hit by a drunk driver in a crash that killed his girlfriend and left him with a serious traumatic brain injury. She spent the next several years monitoring his medications, transporting him to physical and mental health therapy sessions, and advocating for academic accommodations first at his high school and later at college. Combining her medical expertise as a doctor with her personal experience of being a caregiver to a TBI survivor, Dr. Roy-Bornstein has become a vocal advocate for the TBI community. As an Ambassador with the Brain Injury Association of Massachusetts, she speaks regularly to civic groups and businesses about TBI prevention and to high school and college students about the dangers of underage drinking and drunk driving. She also speaks frequently at health care conferences and trauma symposia, educating her medical colleagues in the recognition and management of concussion.

Finally, she uses her skills as an award-winning writer to spread the word about TBI. Her memoir *Crash: A Mother, a Son, and the Journey from Grief to Gratitude* was praised by *Publishers Weekly* as "a remarkable testament exploring one family's journey through a medical nightmare and a new beginning." From her bimonthly health columns in the national newsletter *Pediatrics for Parents* to her essays in *The Boston Globe* and the *Journal of the American Medical Association*, she shares her knowledge, wisdom and her own family's hopeful story of recovery from TBI. Dr. Roy-Bornstein is thrilled to be a part of this book, sending many other TBI stories out into the world.

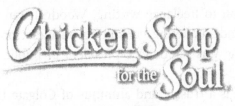

Lee Woodruff and the Bob Woodruff Foundation

As co-author of the New York Times best-selling *In an Instant*, Lee Woodruff garnered critical acclaim for the compelling and humorous chronicle of her family's journey to recovery following her husband Bob's roadside bomb injury in Iraq. Appearing on national television and as keynote speakers since the February 2007 publication of their book, the couple has helped put a face on the serious issue of traumatic brain injury among returning Iraq and Afghanistan war veterans, as well as the millions of Americans who live with this often invisible, but life-changing affliction.

They have founded the Bob Woodruff Foundation to assist post-9/11 injured service members, veterans and their families heal from the physical and silent wounds of war. To date, the non-profit foundation has invested more than $20 million in finding, funding, and shaping innovative programs across the country that are helping veterans successfully integrate back into their communities. Woodruff is a contributing reporter for *CBS This Morning*. Her best-selling book, *Perfectly Imperfect: A Life in Progress*, was followed by her first novel *Those We Love Most*, which became a New York Times Best Seller and won the Washington Irving Book Award for fiction.

A freelance writer, Woodruff has penned numerous personal articles about her family and parenting that have run in magazines such as *Ladies' Home Journal*, *Real Simple*, *Good Housekeeping*, *Redbook*, and *Parade*.

In addition to freelance writing, Woodruff ran her own public relations and marketing consulting business for sixteen years. Before that, she was senior vice president of public relations firm Porter Novelli.

Woodruff is a trustee and alumnus of Colgate University and an avid lover of the Adirondack region. She lives in Westchester County, New York, with her husband and four children. You can learn more at www.leewoodruff.com.

The Bob Woodruff Foundation (BWF), which will receive a contribution for every copy sold of this book, is the non-profit dedicated to ensuring post-9/11 injured service members, veterans and their families are thriving long after they return home. A national organization with grassroots reach, the Bob Woodruff Foundation complements the work of the federal government—diligently navigating the maze of more than 46,000 nonprofits providing services to veterans—finds, funds and shapes innovative programs, and holds them accountable for results. To date, BWF has invested more than $20 million in public education and solutions, reaching more than 1 million service members, support personnel, veterans and their families. The Bob Woodruff Foundation was co-founded in 2006 by award-winning anchor Bob Woodruff and his family, whose own experiences inspired them to help make sure the nation's heroes have access to the highest level of support and resources they deserve, for as long as they need it. For more information about the Bob Woodruff Foundation, please visit bobwoodrufffoundation.org.

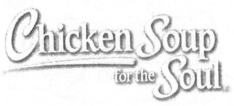

Thank You

We owe huge thanks to all of our contributors. We know that you poured your hearts and souls into the thousands of stories that you shared with us, and ultimately with other people who are recovering from traumatic brain injuries or helping their loved ones do so. As we read and edited these stories, we were truly moved by your experiences and inspired by your great advice. We appreciate your willingness to share these personal, heartfelt stories with our readers. It took extra effort for many of you to write these stories and work with us through the editing process, and we appreciate how unselfishly you have shared your experiences with people who may be new to the TBI community. They will undoubtedly be very grateful to you.

We could only publish a small percentage of the stories that were submitted, but we read every single one and even the ones that do not appear in the book had an influence on us and on the final manuscript. We owe special thanks to Chicken Soup for the Soul's VP and Assistant Publisher D'ette Corona, who read every story, talked to every contributor, and was instrumental in shaping this manuscript. Senior Editor Barbara LoMonaco proofread the manuscript and Editor and Production Manager Kristiana Pastir turned that Word document into a finished book.

We also owe a special thanks to our creative director and book producer, Brian Taylor at Pneuma Books, for his brilliant vision for our covers and interiors.

~Amy Newmark and Carolyn Roy-Bornstein

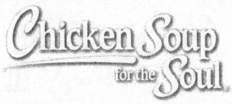

Sharing Happiness, Inspiration, and Wellness

Real people sharing real stories, every day, all over the world. In 2007, *USA Today* named *Chicken Soup for the Soul* one of the five most memorable books in the last quarter-century. With over 100 million books sold to date in the U.S. and Canada alone, more than 200 titles in print, and translations into more than 40 languages, "chicken soup for the soul" is one of the world's best-known phrases.

Today, 21 years after we first began sharing happiness, inspiration and wellness through our books, we continue to delight our readers with new titles, but have also evolved beyond the bookstore, with wholesome and balanced pet food, delicious nutritious comfort food, and a major motion picture in development. Whatever you're doing, wherever you are, Chicken Soup for the Soul is "always there for you™." Thanks for reading!

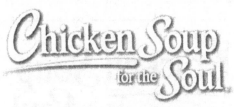

Share with Us

We all have had Chicken Soup for the Soul moments in our lives. If you would like to share your story or poem with millions of people around the world, go to chickensoup.com and click on "Submit Your Story." You may be able to help another reader, and become a published author at the same time. Some of our past contributors have launched writing and speaking careers from the publication of their stories in our books!

We only accept story submissions via our website. They are no longer accepted via mail or fax.

To contact us regarding other matters, please send us an e-mail through webmaster@chickensoupforthesoul.com, or fax or write us at:

Chicken Soup for the Soul
P.O. Box 700
Cos Cob, CT 06807-0700
Fax: 203-861-7194

One more note from your friends at Chicken Soup for the Soul: Occasionally, we receive an unsolicited book manuscript from one of our readers, and we would like to respectfully inform you that we do not accept unsolicited manuscripts and we must discard the ones that appear.

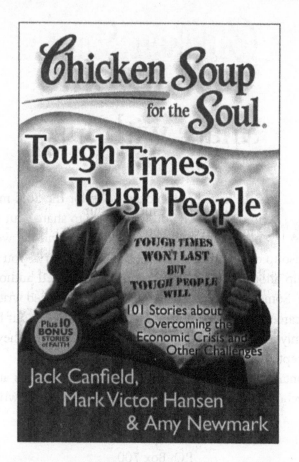

Tough times won't last, but tough people will. Many people have lost money, jobs and/or homes, or made cutbacks. Others have faced life-changing natural disasters, or health and family difficulties. These encouraging and inspirational stories are all about overcoming adversity, pulling together, and finding joy in a simpler life. Stories address downsizing, resolving debt, managing chronic illness, having faith, finding new perspectives, and blessings in disguise.

978-1-935096-35-1

More Inspiration

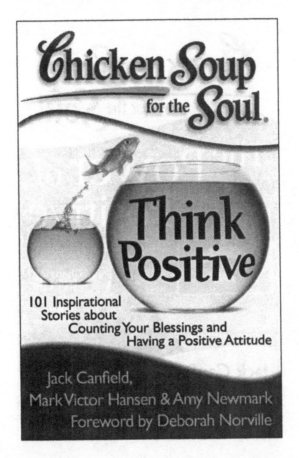

Every cloud has a silver lining. Readers will be inspired by these 101 real-life stories from people just like them, taking a positive attitude to the ups and downs of life, and remembering to be grateful and count their blessings. This book continues Chicken Soup for the Soul's focus on inspiration and hope, and its stories of optimism and faith will encourage readers to stay positive during challenging times and in their everyday lives.

978-1-935096-56-6

and Motivation

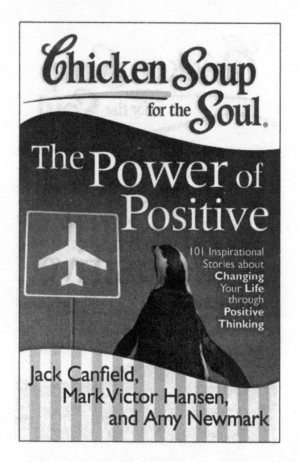

Chicken Soup for the Soul.

The Power of Positive

101 Inspirational Stories about **Changing** Your **Life** through **Positive Thinking**

Jack Canfield, Mark Victor Hansen, and Amy Newmark

Attitude is everything. And this book will uplift and inspire readers with its 101 success stories about the power of positive thinking and how contributors changed their lives, solved problems, or overcame challenges through a positive attitude, counting their blessings, or other epiphanies.

978-1-61159-903-9

Real Stories

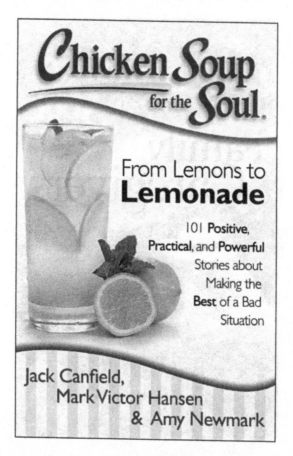

Chicken Soup for the Soul

From Lemons to Lemonade

101 Positive, Practical, and Powerful Stories about Making the Best of a Bad Situation

Jack Canfield,
Mark Victor Hansen
& Amy Newmark

When life hands you lemons... make lemonade! This collection is full of inspiring true stories from others who did just that, and will help you make the best of any bad situation. You will find inspiration, encouragement, and guidance on turning what seemed like a negative into something positive in these 101 sweet stories of success!

978-1-61159-914-5

Overcoming Challenges

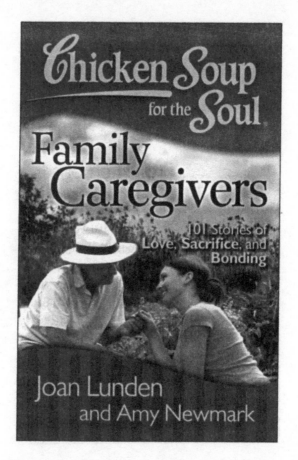

Do you have a family member who requires constant care? You are not alone. This collection offers support and encouragement in its 101 stories for family caregivers of all ages, including the "sandwich" generation caring for a family member while raising their children. With stories by those on the receiving end of the care too. These stories of love, sacrifice, and lessons will inspire and uplift family members making sacrifices to make sure their loved ones are well cared for, whether in their own homes or elsewhere.

978-1-935096-83-2

Sharing Love

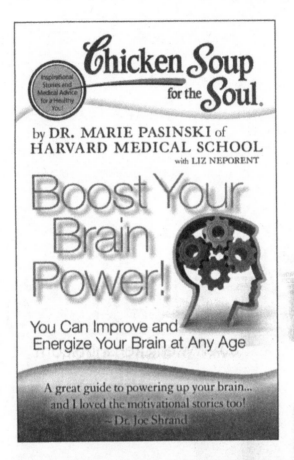

Inspiring Chicken Soup for the Soul stories and accessible leading-edge medical information from Dr. Marie Pasinski of Harvard Medical School. Many people would like to enhance their brainpower and are looking for help to do just that. Others are retraining their brains after traumatic injuries or strokes. Others are looking for ways to keep their brains young and dynamic. This book will fascinate you with stories and useful information on how to improve your own brain.

978-1-935096-86-3

and Great Tips